Chuanan Shen
Editor

Novel Strategies for Critical Burn Care

Translated by Huageng Yuan

Springer

PMPH
PEOPLE'S MEDICAL PUBLISHING HOUSE

Editor
Chuanan Shen
Department of Burns and Plastic Surgery
The Fourth Medical Center of Chinese PLA
Beijing, China

Translated by
Huageng yuan
Beijing, China

ISBN 978-981-92-0324-6 ISBN 978-981-92-0325-3 (eBook)
https://doi.org/10.1007/978-981-92-0325-3

Jointly published with People's Medical Publishing House, PR of China
The print edition is not for sale in China (Mainland). Customers from China (Mainland) please order the print book from: People's Medical Publishing House, PR of China.

This Springer imprint is published by the registered company Springer Nature Singapore Pte Ltd.
The registered company address is: 152 Beach Road, #21-01/04 Gateway East, Singapore 189721, Singapore

Preface

Since its establishment in 1958, modern burn surgery in China has gone through more than six decades of trials and tribulations. Generations of burn specialists have worked diligently, building the specialty from scratch, accumulating specialized knowledge bit by bit, and achieving remarkable accomplishments in basic research, clinical treatment, talent cultivation, and discipline development. I graduated from the Third Military Medical University in 1997 and was fortunate to join the burn surgery team at the former 304th Hospital of the Chinese People's Liberation Army. In my career, I have always aspired to seek truth, act pragmatically, and innovate continuously, all in service of the humanitarian mission of saving lives. In the arduous process of treating critical burns, I have come to understand that "to cure sometimes, to relieve often, to comfort always."

In 2015, we conducted a survey of 2103 cases of large burns admitted within 6 h post-burn from 106 tertiary hospitals in China. The overall cure rate was 77.8%. However, the cure rate was only 36% among 136 patients with a burn size of more than 90% TBSA. To improve the cure rate and foster hope for success, new techniques and methods for burn care were still urgently needed. Based on years of clinical experience and scientific research, I have put forward a series of new concepts and techniques for treating critical burns, which are carefully presented in this book. These new concepts and techniques cover every aspect of burn care, including diagnosis and assessment, shock fluid resuscitation, autologous skin cultivation, wound repair, surgical methods, hemostasis, nutritional support, and reconstructive surgery, forming a new technical system. Since its clinical application 8 years ago, this system has been used to treat more than 500 cases of critical burns, achieving a 98.5% cure rate. Among these were more than 50 extremely critical cases with total burn areas exceeding 90%, such as 100% burns (with 95% third-degree burns), 99.5% third-degree burns with renal failure, 97% third-degree burns with renal failure, and 96% third-degree burns with small intestinal aneurysm bleeding.

As water flows to the lowest places, adapts to its environment, benefits all things, and does not compete, the pioneers of burn medicine created something out of nothing, benefited people far and wide, and selflessly paved the way for others. Their example inspires later generations to inherit, innovate, and persevere. It is my intention to share these insights with burn colleagues and those in the fields of trauma, emergency, and critical care. However, my knowledge and experience are limited. Every time I review this book, I find shortcomings. I sincerely hope that readers will offer their valuable criticisms and suggestions.

Beijing, China Chuanan Shen

Acknowledgments I would like to extend my sincere gratitude to the doctors and nurses on our team. All of the new techniques I proposed have been validated through clinical work—none of this would have been possible without the support of every team member.

I would also like to express my gratitude to Huageng Yuan, translator of the book, for her remarkable sense of responsibility and professionalism. Her invaluable support has played a crucial role in sharing our achievements with a wider audience.

I am deeply grateful to all the patients. They are the source of my innovation, and these new techniques are now helping more and more patients.

Finally, my heartfelt thanks go to People's Medical Publishing House (PMPH) and Kumar Athiappan, production manager, and his team at Springer. It is their efforts that have made it possible for this book to be published and shared with everyone without delay.

Contents

Chapter 1
New Strategies for Burn Diagnosis and Severity Assessment

Chuanan Shen, Wenfeng Cheng, Xinzhu Liu, and Zhaoxing Liu

1.1 Assessment of Burn Size and Depth

1.1.1 Relative and Absolute Size

Customarily, burn size is expressed as the percentage of the surface area burned to the total body surface area (TBSA), which is a relative measurement often estimated with the Rule of Nines and the Rule of Palm [1]. With the Rule of Nines, the head, face, and neck collectively account for approximately 9% of TBSA. With the Rule of Palm, the inner surface of the hand is considered 1% TBSA. This relative method of quantifying burn size has been commonly employed in diagnosing burns and evaluating severity to initiate a proper management for burn patients.

Nevertheless, based on our extensive clinical experience in treating burn patients across a wide spectrum of ages and weights, it has become evident that the absolute burn size holds undeniable importance. This is due to the potentially drastic variations in body surface area among patients of differing ages and weights. For instance, a 30% TBSA burn corresponds to an absolute burn size of approximately 0.19 m^2 in a 3-year-old child weighing 15 kg, whereas it can reach 0.45 m^2 in an adult weighing 50 kg and standing 160 cm tall and 0.67 m^2 in an adult weighing 100 kg and standing 180 cm tall. Consequently, individuals with the same relative burn size may exhibit considerable differences in absolute burn size which plays a crucial role in estimating fluid loss, energy consumption, demand of autologous skin grafts, and biological dressings. Recognizing this variability, the author has developed a new chart for the assessment of burn size and depth (Fig. 1.1).

C. Shen (✉) · W. Cheng · X. Liu · Z. Liu
The Medical Department of Burn and Plastic Surgery, The 4th Medical Center, PLAGH, Beijing, China

C. Shen (ed.), *Novel Strategies for Critical Burn Care*,
https://doi.org/10.1007/978-981-92-0325-3_1

Patient name____________________ Medical Record No.____________________

Mechanism of Injury____

Date/Time of Injury ________________ Date & Time of Admission________________

Height(cm) __________ Weight(kg) __________ Body Surface Area(m^2) __________

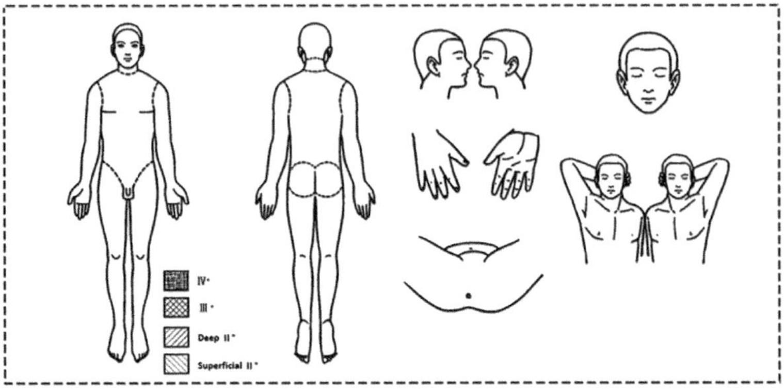

Surface Area (Rule of Nines)

		TBSA%
Head &Neck	Scalp	3
	Face	3
	Neck	3
Trunk	Anterior trunk	13
	Posterior trunk	13
	Perineum	1
Upper extremities	Upper arms	7
	Lower arms	6
	Hands	5
Lower extremities	Buttocks	5
	Thighs	21
	Legs	13
	Feet	7
	Total	100

Relative Burn Size

	Superficial II°	Deep II°	III°	IV°
Scalp				
Face				
Neck				
Anterior trunk				
Posterior trunk				
Perineum				
Upper arms				
Lower arms				
Hands				
Buttocks				
Thighs				
Legs				
Feet				
Total				
Burn Size	%TBSA			

Absolute Burn Size

	Superficial II°	Deep II°	III°	IV°
Scalp				
Face				
Neck				
Anterior trunk				
Posterior trunk				
Perineum				
Upper arms				
Lower arms				
Hands				
Buttocks				
Thighs				
Legs				
Feet				
Total				
Burn Size	m^2			

Fig. 1.1 Diagnosis chart for burn size and depth. (1) Head surface area in children (%) = 9 + (12-age) and surface area of both lower extremities in children (%) = 46-(12-age). (2) For patients aged above 12, body surface area (m^2) = 0.0061 × height (cm) + 0.0128 × weight (kg)-0.1529. (3) For patients≤12 years old, body surface area (m^2) = weight (kg) × 0.035 + 0.1(weight ≤ 30 kg) or body surface area (m^2) = [weight (kg)-30] × 0.02 + 1.05 (weight > 30 kg)

1.1.2 Dynamic Assessment of Burn Size

As treatment progresses, superficial wounds gradually heal through interventions, while deep wounds are also repaired through grafting, resulting in a constantly evolving total wound size. Proportionately, the patient's requirement for fluid, calorie, and nutrition also changes. Now the initial assessment of burn size no longer accurately reflects the ongoing needs of the patient. Considering this, the author proposes the concepts of "initial burn size" and "phased burn size," categorizing the actual and evolving burn sizes at 2, 3, 4, and 5 weeks postburn as phased burn sizes to enhance the precision and adaptability of the care plan.

1.1.3 Dynamic Assessment of Burn Depth

Accurate estimation of burn depth underpins the entire treatment plan and the expectation of patient prognosis. However, in clinical practice, it is extremely difficult to distinguish superficial second-degree wound from deep second-degree wound, as well as deep second-degree wound from third-degree wound in the early stages postburn. The author believes that in clinical settings, dynamic adjustments should be made to the diagnosis as the wound surface features become distinguishable as treatment progresses. Furthermore, burn depth typically does not stay unchanged, with instances of wounds deepening being relatively common in our experience. To enhance the precision and efficacy of burn care, it is imperative to make prompt and dynamic adjustments to the assessment of burn depth as warranted.

1.2 Critical Factors in Burn Severity Assessment

Burn severity assessment constitutes the foundation upon which a series of clinical treatment plans are built, influencing the determination of care interventions, the establishment of monitoring strategies, the decision of whether to transfer the patient, and the prognostic evaluations [2]. As burn care advances, indicators of burn severity increase; as medical team capacity building strengthens, the recovery rate of extensive burns has improved markedly. In order to align with the evolving landscape of this medical specialty, it is imperative to adapt and refine the classification criteria for assessing burn severity.

1.2.1 Burn Size

The authors conducted a study analyzing the treatment of 2103 patients with large and extensive burns admitted to the burn departments of 106 tertiary hospitals in China within 6 h post-injury and found that [3]:

The recovery rate was about 85% in 30% ~ 39% TBSA and 40 ~ 49% TBSA burns
About 75% in 50 ~ 59% TBSA and 60 ~ 69% TBSA burns
About 60% in 70 ~ 79% TBSA and 80 ~ 89% TBSA burns
Notably, plummeted to below 40% once the burn size surpassed 90% (Table 1.1)

Based on this, our team proposed modified criteria for burn severity classification:

- Severe: 30 ~ 49% TBSA
- Extremely severe: 50 ~ 69% TBSA
- Critical: 70%~ 89% TBSA
- Extremely critical: 90 ~ 100% TBSA

With the proposed criteria, the recovery rate of the 2103 patients can be represented as in Table 1.2.

The Analytic Hierarchy Process found that in 30–49% TBSA burns, though the recovery rate reached 90% in young and middle-aged patients aged 15 ~ 59, it dropped to 55% in the elders aged 60 and above (Table 1.3). Therefore, considering 30% TBSA as the threshold of severe burns is believed to be in line with actual treatment level.

1.2.2 Burn Index

In the context of large or extensive burns of equivalent size, varying depths of burn injuries present diverse challenges in treatment. Researchers have utilized the burn index (BI) as a metric to assess the severity of burns [4]. Our study of the 2103 burn

Table 1.1 Recovery profile of 2103 burn patients from 106 hospitals

	Sum (n = 2103)		
Burn size (%TBSA)	Total	Recovered	Recovery rate
30 ~ 39	916	801	87.45%
40 ~ 49	390	322	82.56%
50 ~ 59	251	187	74.50%
60 ~ 69	165	129	78.18%
70 ~ 79	135	86	63.70%
80 ~ 89	110	63	57.27%
90 ~ 100	136	49	36.03%

TBSA total body surface area

Table 1.2 Recovery profile of the 2103 burn patients represented with the proposed criteria

		Sum ($n = 2103$)		
Burn severity	Burn size (%TBSA)	Total	Recovered	Recovery rate
Severe	30 ~ 49	1306	1123	85.99%
Extremely severe	50 ~ 69	416	316	75.96%
Critical	70 ~ 89	245	149	60.82%
Extremely critical	90 ~ 100	136	49	36.03%

patients revealed that the mortality rate of burn patients escalated with increasing BI values, rising from 0.18% for BI 15 ~ 24 to 2.39% for BI 25 ~ 34, 9.18% for BI 35 ~ 44 and to more than 71.15% for BI ≥75. Kaplan-Meier survival curves demonstrate statistically significant differences in mortality rates among different BI groups (log-rank test, $\chi^2 = 1097.430$, $P < 0.01$) (see Fig. 1.2).

To better understand the relation between BI and treatment outcomes, the receiver operator characteristic curve (ROC) was utilized to assess the sensitivity and specificity of different BI values. The results revealed a notable increase in mortality rates when BI reaches 41. The maximum Youden Index evaluating BI's performance in prognostic assessment was calculated at 0.76, with a sensitivity of 0.90 and a specificity of 0.86 (Fig. 1.3).

The ROC curve analysis yielded an AUC of 0.94 (95% CI: 0.93–0.95), indicating that BI can serve as a reliable indicator for predicting treatment outcomes of large and extensive burns (Fig. 1.4). A subsequent multivariate logistic regression analysis considered factors such as the patient's gender, age, time elapsed since injury, prehospital emergency care, burn etiology, and the presence of inhalation injuries. The results indicated that patients with a BI ≥ 41 faced a mortality risk 10.93 times higher than those with a BI < 41.

1.2.3 Age

The prevalence of severely burned elderly individuals is on the rise in tandem with the aging demographics of society [5]. As bodily tissues and organs undergo the aging process, there is a concomitant decline in physiological and reserve functions. Elderly patients commonly present with chronic or previously undiagnosed subclinical conditions that may exacerbate outcomes post-injury. The interplay of these diverse factors renders the post-injury progression, disease prognosis, and treatment outcomes of elderly burn patients distinct from those of their younger counterparts. In the 1980s, researchers utilized a combination of age and the size of third-degree burns to predict mortality rates, underscoring the significant impact of age on the prognosis of severely burned individuals. The analysis of the data presented in Table 1.3 shows that the recovery rate (55%) for 30% ~ 49% TBSA burns in elderly burn patients is lower than the recovery rate (69%) for 70 ~ 89% TBSA burns in young and middle-aged patients. Furthermore, elderly patients with burn size

Table 1.3 Recovery rate of 2103 cases of large and extensive burns from 106 hospitals across different age groups

	≤14 years old ($n = 435$)			15 ~ 59 years old ($n = 1410$)			≥60 years old ($n = 258$)		
Burn size (%TBSA)	Total	Recovered	Recovery rate	Total	Recovered	Recovery rate	Total	Recovered	Recovery rate
30 ~ 49	369	323	87.53%	791	719	90.90%	146	81	55.48%
50 ~ 69	50	37	74.00%	307	252	82.08%	59	27	45.76%
70 ~ 89	10	5	50.00%	194	134	69.07%	41	10	24.39%
90 ~ 100	6	2	33.33%	118	47	39.83%	12	0	0.00%

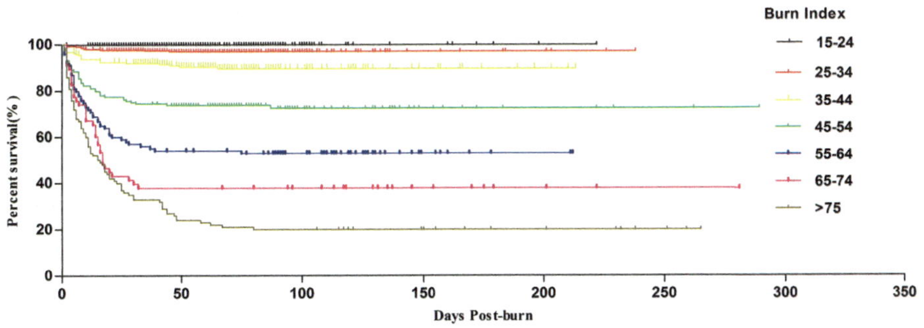

Fig. 1.2 Kaplan-Meier survival curves of different BI groups

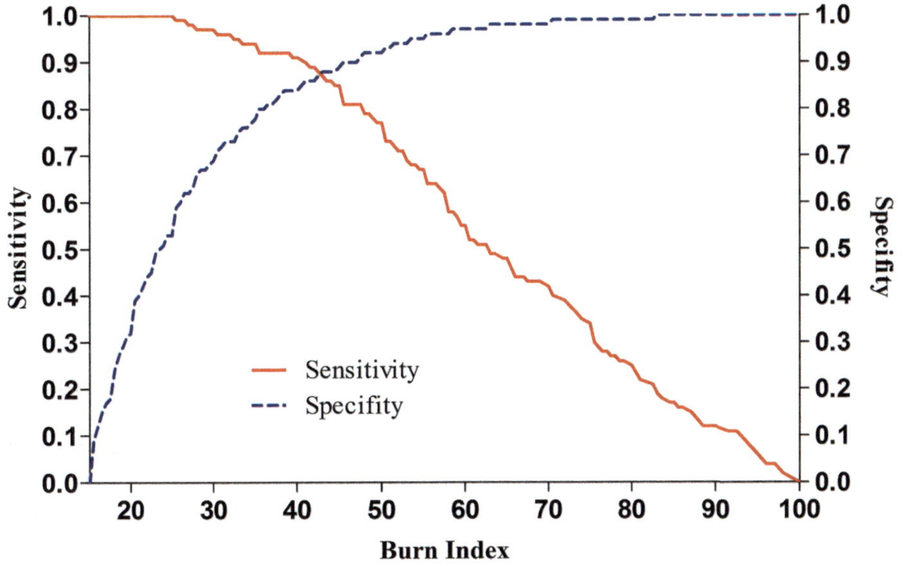

Fig. 1.3 Analysis of the optimal cutoff point of BI in predicting prognosis of patients with large and extensive burns

exceeding 90% TBSA exhibit a mortality rate of 100%. Based on these findings, the authors propose a classification criterion for burn severity in the elderly population: 30 ~ 49% TBSA should be classified as critical burns and ≥ 50% TBSA extremely critical burns.

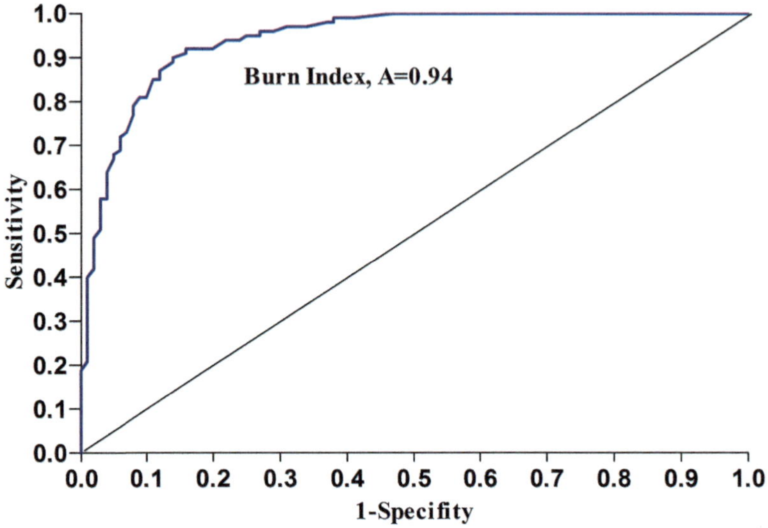

Fig. 1.4 Receiver operating characteristic curve for using BI in evaluating the prognosis of patients with large and extensive burns. *BI* burn index, *AUC* area under the curve

1.2.4 Diabetes

It has been found in clinical work that when a diabetic patient sustains large or extensive burns, the treatment will encounter increased difficulties. An analysis of the 2103 cases of large and extensive burns found that the recovery rate of 101 diabetic patients was significantly lower than that of nondiabetic patients with equivalent burn sizes, yet similar to that of nondiabetic patients with larger burn sizes of the next level (Table 1.4). Based on this, the authors believe that burn severity classification for diabetic patient should be differentiated from that of patients without underlying diseases. The authors suggest a tailored classification system to support better management for diabetic patients: 30 ~ 49% TBSA should be classified as extremely severe burn, 50 ~ 69% TBSA critical burns, and ≥70% TBSA extremely critical burns.

1.2.5 Procalcitonin

Procalcitonin (PCT), the pro-peptide of calcitonin, comprises 116 amino acids and possesses a molecular weight of approximately 13 kD. It consists of 57 amino acids at the N-terminus, premature calcitonin, and katacalcin. Physiologically, PCT is predominantly produced by thyroid C-cells and undergoes proteolytic cleavage to yield calcitonin, which plays a pivotal role in regulating calcium metabolism. The serum concentration of PCT in healthy individuals is below detection limit

Table 1.4 Analysis of the recovery rate of 101 diabetic patients with large and extensive burns from 106 hospitals

Burn size (%TBSA)	Diabetic patient (n = 101)			Nondiabetic patient (n = 2002)			Total (n = 2103)		
	Total	Recovered	Recovery rate	Total	Recovered	Recovery rate	Total	Recovered	Recovery rate
30 ~ 49	51	37	72.55%	1255	1086	86.53%	1306	1123	85.99%
50 ~ 69	22	13	59.09%	394	303	76.90%	416	316	75.96%
70 ~ 89	20	7	35.00%	225	142	63.11%	245	149	60.82%
90 ~ 100	8	0	0.00%	128	49	38.28%	136	49	36.03%

(<0.01 ng/m) [6]. In the presence of severe bacterial infection, the body's innate immune system recognizes the pathogen associated molecular pattern (PAMP) carried in lipopolysaccharide on pathogen surface, triggering a systemic inflammatory response. Upon exposure to endotoxins and inflammatory cytokines, the expression of the calcitonin gene is upregulated in cells across various tissues other than in the thyroid, resulting in a substantial production of PCT. However, these extra-thyroidal tissues lack the requisite specific proteolytic enzymes for PCT cleavage, resulting in release of uncleaved PCT in significant quantities, consequently elevating PCT levels in the plasma. Mitochondria exhibit structural similarities to bacterial cells and represent the sole organelles in cells that have their own DNA apart from the nucleus. In the presence of certain noninfectious conditions such as severe trauma, shock, and major surgery, mitochondria from disintegrated and necrotic cells rupture, releasing damage-associated molecular patterns (DAMPs) that elicit similar host responses to PAMPs. Theses DAMPs can also be recognized by patter recognition receptors (PRRs) on the surface of immune cells, provoking a systemic inflammatory response reminiscent of a severe infection and resulting in an elevation of PCT levels [7].

The first 48-h post-burn is also known as the shock stage during which severe infection generally does not occur, while a marked increase of circulating PCT is often observed. Our team retrospectively analyzed the data of 139 patients with extremely severe burns (≥50% TBSA), investigating the contributing factors to elevated PCT levels and their potential implications for guiding treatment decisions [8]. The analysis found that among the cohort, though 72 individuals (51.8%) manifested a significant elevation in PCT levels (≥2 ng/mL) during the shock stage, despite the absence of obvious infection cues—neither clinical manifestations nor positive diagnostic findings—suggesting that PCT elevations during the early post-burn period were not infection-induced changes. The correlation analysis showed that serum PCT level was positively correlated with burn size ($r = 0.440$, $P < 0.001$) and burn index ($r = 0.463$, $P < 0.001$). Furthermore, PCT levels during the burn shock stage also exhibited positive correlations with age, delay in resuscitation, presence of inhalation injury, Acute Physiology and Chronic Health Evaluation II (APACHE II) scores, and Sepsis-related Organ Failure Assessment (SOFA) scores, suggesting that its increase is caused by a combination of various noninfectious factors such as skin injury, shock, stress response, and organ impairments (Table 1.5). Moreover, escalated PCT levels during the shock stage were also positively correlated with mortality rate, which rose to 30% when PCT surpassed 3 ng/mL and reached 50% when PCT exceeded 5 ng/mL. Deceased patients exhibited significantly higher peak PCT value in the shock stage than survivors [11.16 (3.57–22.95) vs. 1.48 (0.64–4.32), $P < 0.001$]. The area under the ROC curve (AUC) for predicting mortality stood at 0.788, with an optimal threshold of 5.4 ng/mL, offering a sensitivity of 70.4% and a specificity of 81.3% (Table 1.6 and Fig. 1.5).

After the shock stage, the granulation barrier on the wound surface has not yet been established, the organ functions have not fully recovered from the severe shock, and substantial necrotic tissues and exudates have accumulated on the wound surface, all providing favorable conditions for bacterial colonization and subsequent

Table 1.5 Correlation analysis between serum PCT levels and part of the factors affecting the severity of extremely severe burns

	PCT-SP		PCT-IP	
Factors	*r*	*P*	*r*	*P*
Age	−0.241	0.004	−0.068	0.430
Gender (female)	−0.199	0.019	0.239	0.005
Etiology of burns				
Flame	0.198	0.019	0.179	0.041
Hot liquid	−0.066	0.437	−0.078	0.297
Chemicals	0.167	0.086	0.133	0.125
Burn-blast	0.211	0.012	0.172	0.055
Burn size	0.440	<0.001	0.452	<0.001
Burn index	0.463	<0.001	0.524	<0.001
Grades of inhalation injury				
Mild	0.169	0.081	0.124	0.146
Moderate	0.341	<0.001	0.332	<0.001
Severe	0.513	<0.001	0.498	<0.001
Resuscitation delay	0.245	0.004	0.241	0.004
APACHE II score	0.349	<0.001	0.339	<0.001
SOFA score	0.516	<0.001	0.549	<0.001

PCT-SP peak value of procalcitonin in the shock stage, *PCT-IP* peak value of procalcitonin in the infection stage, *SOFA* sepsis-related organ failure assessment, *APACHE* acute physiology and chronic health evaluation

Table 1.6 Correlation analysis between serum PCT levels and mortality in patients with extremely severe burns

PCT-SP				PCT-IP			
Concentration / (ng·mL^{-1})	Total cases	Death cases	Death rate	concentration / (ng·mL^{-1})	Total cases	Death cases	Death rate
<0.50	23	1	4.3%	<0.50	15	0	0
0.50 ~ 0.99	23	2	8.7%	0.50 ~ 0.99	25	0	0
1.00 ~ 1.99	21	1	4.8%	1.00 ~ 1.99	31	1	3.2%
2.00 ~ 4.99	29	4	13.8%	2.00 ~ 4.99	20	2	10.0%
5.00 ~ 9.99	16	5	31.3%	5.00 ~ 9.99	17	4	23.5%
10.00 ~ 19.99	12	6	50.0%	10.00 ~ 19.99	9	4	33.3%
≥20.00	15	8	53.3%	≥20.00	22	17	77.3%
r		0.395		*r*		0.584	
P		<0.001		*P*		<0.001	

PCT-SP peak value of procalcitonin in the shock stage, *PCT-IP* peak value of procalcitonin in the infection stage

infections. Therefore, the subsequent stage is commonly recognized as the infection stage. An analysis showed that 61.8% of patients with significantly elevated PCT levels (≥2 ng/m) during the infection stage developed severe systemic infection. PCT levels during the infection stage also exhibited significant correlations with

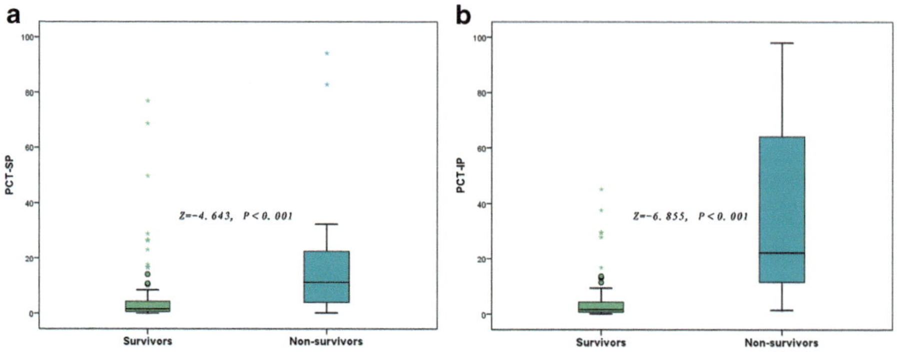

Fig. 1.5 Comparison of serum PCT levels between survivors and non-survivors

APACHE II and SOFA scores. Elevated peak PCT levels are indicative of increased susceptibility to sepsis, multi-organ failure, and death. Notably, the peak PCT levels in the infection stage among the non-survivors significantly exceeded those of survivors [22.29 (9.34–64.23) vs. 1.59 (0.77–4.43), $P < 0.001$]. The AUC reached 0.926, with an optimal prognostic threshold of 8.5 ng/mL, offering a sensitivity of 85.2% and a specificity of 88.4%, respectively (Table 1.6 and Fig. 1.5).

A multivariate logistic regression analysis was conducted to further investigate the prognostic variables and showed that the peak value of PCT over 5.4 ng/mL (OR = 5.33) during the shock stage and that over 8.5 ng/mL (OR = 14.49) during the infection stage predict a higher risk of death. It is suggested that PCT can serve as an effective biomarker for severity assessment and outcome prediction for burn patients. PCT levels exceeding these thresholds indicate an increased risk of poor outcomes which should alert physicians to reassess and optimize treatment strategies accordingly.

References

1. Colson CD, Alberto EC, Milestone ZP, et al. EasyTBSA as a method for calculating total body surface area burned: a validation study. Emerg Med J. 2023;40(4):279–84.
2. Fadeyibi IO, Jewo PI, Saalu LC, Akinola OI, Fabamwo O, Ademiluyi SA. Burn severity and post-burn infertility in men. Burns. 2010;36(3):367–71.
3. Cheng W, Shen C, Zhao D, et al. The epidemiology and prognosis of patients with massive burns: a multicenter study of 2483 cases. Burns. 2019;45(3):705–16.
4. Zhang JX, Ahmed SN, Pangli H, Papp A. Predicting and estimating burn outcomes: an institutional analysis of 4622 cases. J Burn Care Res. 2022;43(6):1426–33.
5. Edgar DW, Homer L, Phillips M, Gurfinkel R, Rea S, Wood FM. The influence of advancing age on quality of life and rate of recovery after treatment for burn. Burns. 2013;39(6):1067–72. https://doi.org/10.1016/j.burns.2013.05.017.
6. Parli SE, Trivedi G, Woodworth A, et al. Procalcitonin: usefulness in acute care surgery and trauma. Surg Infect. 2018;19(2):131–6.

7. Ren B, Zou G, Huang Y, et al. Serum levels of HSP70 and other DAMP proteins can aid in patient diagnosis after traumatic injury. Cell Stress Chaperones. 2016;21(4):677–86.
8. Liu Z, Li D, Liu X, Zhang B, Zang Y, Ma J, Zhang W, Niu Y, Shen C. Elevated serum procalcitonin to predict severity and prognosis of extensive burns. J Investig Surg. 2022;35(7):1510–8. https://doi.org/10.1080/08941939.2022.2073489. Epub 2022 May 15.

Chapter 2
New Formulas for Burn Resuscitation

Chuanan Shen and Xinzhu Liu

Shock is one of the severest complications in the early stage postburn. Though the mortality rate of extensive burns during the shock stage has decreased significantly due to the constant advance in burn care, delayed resuscitation along with other unstable patient conditions such as ischemia-hypoxic injuries and renal function impairment during burn shock would pose formidable challenges to the subsequent treatment [1, 2]. Therefore, assiduous management to help the patient get through the shock stage smoothly is the first key link in a series of successful treatment of extensive burns.

2.1 Management of Burn Resuscitation

Extensive burns cause severe damage to the "two barriers" in body fluid regulation: First, the skin on the body surface is badly damaged, resulting in grave loss of plasma-like fluid, and second, increased vascular permeability allows large quantities of intravascular fluid to extravasate into the interstitium [3]. The loss and extravasation of fluid lead to a rapid decline in circulating blood volume and in perfusion to tissues and organs, inducing ischemia-hypoxic injuries and the release of inflammatory mediators, which, in turn, aggravates tissue injury [4].

2.1.1 The Key to Burn Shock Prevention and Treatment Lies in "Resuscitation as Early as Possible"

In treating patients with extensive burns either at the site or in the emergency room, it is critical to start fluid resuscitation as soon as possible to get the patient through the shock stage and reduce the risk of complications [5]. Our team found that in

C. Shen (✉) · X. Liu
The Medical Department of Burn and Plastic Surgery, The 4th Medical Center, PLAGH, Beijing, China

C. Shen (ed.), *Novel Strategies for Critical Burn Care*,
https://doi.org/10.1007/978-981-92-0325-3_2

miniature pig models of burns (50% TBSA, III degree), it is notable that from half hour postburn HCT and hemoconcentration increased, cardiac output markedly decreased, tissue perfusion declined, and urine output reduced, with a darkened color of the urine and even gross hematuria. Notably, these injuries can be alleviated by correcting circulating blood volume through fluid administration as soon as possible.

2.1.2 *Tenfold Formulas for Burn Resuscitation*

Before the transfer of severely burned patients to a burn center where specialized and precise care is provided, a quick and reliable calculation of fluid requirements would greatly aid the efforts of the emergency team and the stabilization of the patient. In our experience, such needs can be well addressed with two fast formulas concluded by the author. The first is the tenfold formula for adult patients: [fluid infusion in ml/h =10 × %TBSA] (Table 2.1), and the second is the tenfold formula for pediatric patients: [fluid infusion in ml/h =10 × body weight (kg)] (Table 2.2). The two formulas are devised for burn resuscitation in the first 8 h post-burn in emergency scenarios where specialized care cannot be accessed. Crystalloid is the first choice if accessible [6]. After successful transfer of the patient to a burn center, more accurate fluid administration begins. Several specialized formulas provide elaborate calculations of fluid requirements during the first 24 h and first 8 h postburn. For example, the commonly used "304 formula" by the burn center at the Chinese People's Liberation Army General Hospital

Table 2.1 Comparison between the "tenfold" formula for adult burn patients and other commonly used resuscitation formulas for the estimation of fluid requirements for an average adult (70 kg) in the first 8 h postburn

	Fluid requirement (mL/h)			
Burn size (%TBSA)	The tenfold formula	The 304 formula	The formula by the Third Military Medical University in China	The Evans formula
30	300	360	322	388
50	500	519	453	563
70	700	676	584	738
90	900	834	716	913
Ratio (tenfold formula: other)				
30	–	0.83	0.93	0.77
50	–	0.96	1.10	0.89
70	–	1.04	1.20	0.95
90	–	1.08	1.26	0.99

The 304 formula: [%TBSA × weight (kg) × (0.9 + 0.9) +2000] mL
The Third Military Medical University formula: [%TBSA × weight (kg) × (1.0 + 0.5) +2000] mL
The Evans formula: [%TBSA × weight (kg) × (1 + 1) +2000] mL
The tenfold formula for adult burn patients: (%TBSA×10) mL

Table 2.2 Comparison between the "tenfold" formula for pediatric burn patients and the fluid formula for children by China Burn Association (CBA) for the estimation of fluid requirements in the first 8 h postburn

			Fluid formula for children by CBA (ml/ h)			
Age (years)	Weight (kg)	Tenfold (mL/h)	30%TBSA	50%TBSA	70%TBSA	90%TBSA
1	10	100	100 ~ 131	125 ~ 156	150 ~ 181	175 ~ 206
2	12	120	120 ~ 157	150 ~ 187	180 ~ 218	210 ~ 248
5	18	180	115 ~ 171	154 ~ 210	194 ~ 250	233 ~ 290
7	22	220	140 ~ 209	189 ~ 257	237 ~ 306	285 ~ 354

The weight (kg) of pediatric patients can be estimated according to the following:
3 ~ 12 months: [age (month) + 9]/2
1 ~ 6 years old: age (year) × 2 + 8
7 ~ 12 years old: [age (year) × 7–5]/2
Fluid formula for children by CBA:
<2 years old: [%TBSA× weight (kg) × 2.0 + (100 ~ 150) × weight (kg)] mL
2~12 years old: [%TBSA× weight (kg) × 1.75 + (50 ~ 100) × weight (kg)] mL
The tenfold formula for pediatric burn patients: [weight (kg) × 10] mL

(PLAGH) stated that the volume an average adult patient requires in the first 24 h is 0.9 mL of colloid and 0.9 mL of crystalloid per percent burn per kilogram body weight plus 2000 ml of D5W [%TBSA × body weight × (0.9 mL crystalloid +0.9 mL colloid) + 2000 mL D5W] [7]. The formula recommends giving the first half of the total volume in the first 8 h and the second half in the following 16 h; fluid needs in the second 24 h are calculated as 0.7 mL of colloid and 0.7 mL of electrolyte per percent burn per kilogram body weight plus 2000 ml of D5W [%TBSA × body weight × (0.7 mL colloid +0.7 mL electrolyte) + 2000 mL D5W]. As for pediatric patients, maintenance fluid requirement is the majority part of their total fluid requirement which can be slightly adjusted following the individual's response to therapy. Practically, there are many factors affecting fluid requirements, such as burn depth, patient age, whether inhalation injury is present, and whether resuscitation is delayed, plasma administered, a suspension bed used or an escharotomy performed, etc. [8]. Therefore, the specialized formulas only provide some guidance, and the volume of fluid to be actually administered should be adjusted according to the individual patient's response to therapy and results of various tests and measurements.

With easy memorization and rapid computation, "tenfold formulas" are intended for emergency settings to enhance the preparedness of emergency personnel, particularly those lacking specialized expertise in burn care, thereby facilitating more assured and effective burn rescue operations. The formulas provide reliable estimations, as evidenced in Tables 2.1 and 2.2, where the hourly fluid requirements in the first 8 h, calculated with the "tenfold" formula, closely align with the results from other specialized formulas.

2.1.3 Medications

Attention should be paid to the administration of medications during burn shock resuscitation. These medications primarily encompass oxygen-derived free radical scavengers such as vitamin C and mannitol, edema-alleviating agents such as hormones and diuretics, renal tubule-protecting urinary alkalizers like sodium bicarbonate, and anti-infectives like antibiotics. In addition, patients with underlying conditions such as hypertension, diabetes, and hypothyroidism, among others, should receive tailored treatment with antihypertensive medications, anticoagulants, hypoglycemics, or thyroid hormone replacement therapy as appropriate [9].

2.1.4 Wounds

In this session, the authors would like to emphasize prompt escharotomy in circumferential burns where compromised circulation or respiration occurs. During this procedure, complete hemostasis must be achieved, and timely replenishment of red blood cells should be ensured when necessary [10].

2.1.5 Tubes

The management of extensive burns during the initial phase necessitates a systematic approach with strict adherence to sterilization protocols. Procedures such as insertion of invasive tubes such as IV lines, catheters, or tracheostomy tubes require extreme caution. When feasible, resuscitation fluids can be administered via peripheral veins accessed through unburned skin using a large-bore trocar. Other invasive techniques such as arterial monitoring, Pulse Contour Cardiac Output (PiCCO), and Swan-Ganz catheters should be reserved for cases where they offer clear advantages over less invasive measures. Patients with tracheostomies require secure fixation of the tracheal cannula to prevent displacement. Monitoring for neck edema is essential, with adjustments made to fixation straps as needed to maintain cannula position securely.

2.2 Key Signs and Parameters in Monitoring Fluid Resuscitation

2.2.1 Vital Signs

Careful measurement of vital signs is integral to the management of critically ill patients, and the concept is unequivocally applicable in the context of burn shock resuscitation. Either excessive or insufficient fluid replacement leads to alterations in the patient's consciousness level, heart rate, and respiratory rate. Clinical manifestations such as heightened irritability, increased heart rate, clear breath sounds, and oliguria are often indicative of insufficient fluid infusion rate.

2.2.2 Urine Output

Currently, urine output remains the gold standard for assessing the adequacy of burn shock resuscitation. It directly reflects renal perfusion and microcirculation, thereby offering insights into the overall status of effective circulating volume and hemodynamics. Generally, an hourly urine output ranging between 0.5 and 1.0 mL per kilogram of an individual's body weight is considered acceptable for adult patients undergoing resuscitation. And clinically, the urine output for reference can be calculated as follows: ① for young and middle-aged patients, the hourly urine output (mL) = body weight (kg) × 1.0, and ② for pediatric and geriatric patients, the hourly urine output (mL) = body weight (kg) × 0.8. In the event of excessive or insufficient urine output, the infusion rate needs to be timely adjusted to prevent complications such as pulmonary edema, renal impairment, or even shock. Caution should be exercised with treatment decisions if diuretics are administered, for an increase in urine output may not necessarily signify excessive fluid resuscitation, while a decrease surely indicates either renal injury or insufficient fluid replacement.

2.2.3 Blood Tests

2.2.3.1 Hematocrit

Patients with large burns invariably endure erythrocyte damage in the initial stage after the injury. An increased hematocrit (HCT) during the shock stage is a definite indicator of a reduced effective circulating volume, whereas a decreased HCT should alert the physician to the possibility of over-resuscitation or hidden blood loss, which could emanate from sources such as wound bleeding after escharotomy or gastrointestinal bleeding.

2.2.3.2 Blood Lactate

Blood lactate level reflects the microcirculation and oxygen supply to tissues. An elevated lactate value indicates compromised perfusion and a disruption in aerobic metabolism, which are often warning signs for insufficient resuscitation.

2.2.4 Invasive Monitoring

2.2.4.1 Central Venous Pressure (CVP)

During the resuscitation period, a low central venous pressure (CVP) is not a reliable indicator of insufficient resuscitation, and to blindly "push" the CVP might inadvertently precipitate over-resuscitation; however, an elevated CVP is reliable in indicating either excessive fluid replacement or increased pulmonary vascular resistance.

2.2.4.2 Invasive Blood Pressure

Following severe burns, the extensive loss of plasma-like fluid through the wound surface results in increased permeability of the vascular wall. This permits a massive leakage of intravascular fluid into extravascular spaces, precipitating a rapid decline in effective circulating volume, a marked decrease in cardiac stroke volume, an increase in HCT, and a decrease in urine output. However, with the body's compensatory mechanisms, such as an increase in peripheral vascular resistance (PVR), the blood pressure can be temporarily maintained. Consequently, invasive blood pressure monitoring during burn resuscitation may not present significant utility and could potentially increase the risk of infection.

2.2.4.3 Pulmonary Artery Wedge Pressure and Stroke Volume

Widely used in the field of critical care, PiCCO and Swan-Ganz catheters provide direct quantification of pulmonary artery wedge pressure, stroke volume, and other parameters. The authors believe that for patients with limited burn size, resuscitation can be informed by the aforementioned indices such as vital signs, urine output, and blood lactate levels. Only for extremely extensive burns with cardiopulmonary and renal dysfunction, or even renal failure, situations where the accurate quantification of fluid load becomes challenging, the deployment of PiCCO or Swan-Ganz catheters could be recommended. Unfortunately, the prognosis for such patients is typically unfavorable.

References

1. Shen C, et al. Establishment and application of the tenfold rehydration formula for emergency resuscitation of adult patients after extensive burns. Zhonghua Shao Shang Yu Chuang Mian Xiu Fu Za Zhi. 2022;38(3):236–41.
2. Shen C, et al. Establishment and application of the ten-fold rehydration formula for emergency resuscitation of pediatric patients after extensive burns. Zhonghua Shao Shang Yu Chuang Mian Xiu Fu Za Zhi. 2023;39(1):59–64.
3. Gutowska I, et al. The extent of burn injury significantly affects serum micro- and macroelement concentrations in patients on the first day of hospitalisation. Nutrients. 2022;14(20)
4. Anipindi M, Kacarow J, Bitetto D. Systemic capillary leak syndrome (SCLS) presentation in patients receiving anti-cancer treatments. Cureus. 2023;15(4):e38335.
5. Tan L, et al. The new Nano-resuscitation solution (TPP-MR) attenuated myocardial injury in Hemorrhagic shock rats by inhibiting Ferroptosis. Int J Nanomedicine. 2024;19:7567–83.
6. Cappuyns L, et al. Review of burn resuscitation: is Plasmalyte® a comparable alternative to ringer's lactate? J Burn Care Res. 2023;44(1):81–6.
7. Shen C. Preliminary discussion on the prevention and treatment of shock after severe burns. Zhonghua Shao Shang Yu Chuang Mian Xiu Fu Za Zhi. 2022;38(1):9–12.
8. Davis BN, et al. Acute Burn Care. Plast Reconstr Surg. 2024;153(4):804e–23e.
9. Cartotto R, et al. American burn association clinical practice guidelines on burn shock resuscitation. J Burn Care Res. 2024;45(3):565–89.
10. James AJ, et al. The anatomy of Grayson's ligament and Cleland's ligament: the basis of digit Escharotomy for circumferential full thickness burns of the fingers. Ann Plast Surg. 2025;95(1):51–3.

Chapter 3
New Techniques for Burn Wound Care

Chuanan Shen, Bohan Zhang, Xinzhu Liu, Huping Deng, Jianhua Cai, Dongjie Li, Tianjun Sun, and Dawei Li

3.1 Autologous Skin Graft: In vivo Cultivation

[Background]

The greatest barrier to successful treatment of extensive burns is the paucity of autologous skin. The optimal utilization of residual autologous skin has long been a pivotal concern in burn surgery. Various grafting techniques, such as microskin grafting, intermingled autologous and allogeneic skin grafting, the Meek technique, postage-stamp skin grafting, and mesh skin grafting, rely on small autologous skin grafts to provide coverage for large wounds. Among them, microskin grafting exhibits the highest expansion ratio, reaching up to 1:15, followed by the Meek technique with a ratio of up to 1:9 [1, 2]. Our study, analyzing the treatment outcomes of 2103 patients with large and extensive burns from 106 burn centers at tertiary hospitals across China, revealed that when the total burn size exceeded 90% TBSA, the overall recovery rate stood at a mere 36% [3]. A significant contributing factor to this persists as the severe limitation in the availability of autologous skin, a challenge that has not been addressed through the abovementioned techniques, which were designed to improve the expansion instead of the availability of autologous skin.

As the proverb suggests, "one cannot make bricks without straw"; to cultivate an ample supply of autologous skin grafts will undoubtedly address the challenge at its root. Advances in in vitro cell culture have enabled the cultivation and clinical application of cultured epithelial autografts (CEAs) [4]. While previously prevalent in developed regions of Europe and America, the utilization of these cell sheets has waned due to concerns over extended culture cycles, costliness, thinness, susceptibility to posttransplantation infections, and limited efficacy [5]. In light of these

C. Shen (✉) · B. Zhang · X. Liu · H. Deng · J. Cai · D. Li · T. Sun · D. Li
The Medical Department of Burn and Plastic Surgery, The 4th Medical Center, PLAGH, Beijing, China

C. Shen (ed.), *Novel Strategies for Critical Burn Care*,
https://doi.org/10.1007/978-981-92-0325-3_3

limitations, there has been a shift toward exploring alternative approaches. Based on Meek microskin grafting, we introduce a new concept and technique for in vivo cultivation of autologous skin grafts, which has been confirmed to be efficacious in addressing the paucity of autologous skin and yielding favorable outcomes in the treatment of extensive burns.

[Cultivation Protocol]

1. Fabrication of Meek microskin grafts: A proper amount of split-thickness autologous skin (0.3 mm thick) from unaffected areas of the injured patient is harvested using an electric dermatome, washed thrice with normal saline, and then made into Meek microskin grafts at an expansion ratio of 1:4.
2. Grafting procedure: The burned extremity is excised to the dermal or deep fascial layer (Fig. 3.1a). Subsequently, the prepared Meek microskin grafts are meticulously applied to the freshly excised wound bed, specifically on the flexor surface in the anterior antebrachial or brachial region, or the posterior crural region (Fig. 3.1b).
3. Post-grafting dressing change: Dressings are first changed on the third day post-grafting and every other day subsequently. Approximately 10 days later, full epithelialization of the interstices in the Meek microskin grafts is achieved, and cultivation of more autologous skin grafts is accomplished (Fig. 3.1c).
4. Sequential cultivation process: A proper amount of the newly cultivated autologous skin is harvested with an electric dermatome (Fig. 3.1d). A quarter of these grafts are allocated for repeated fabrication of 1:4 Meek grafts, of which 1/4 are back-grafted to the donor site on the flexor surface and the rest 3/4 are reserved for wound coverage in other parts of the body.

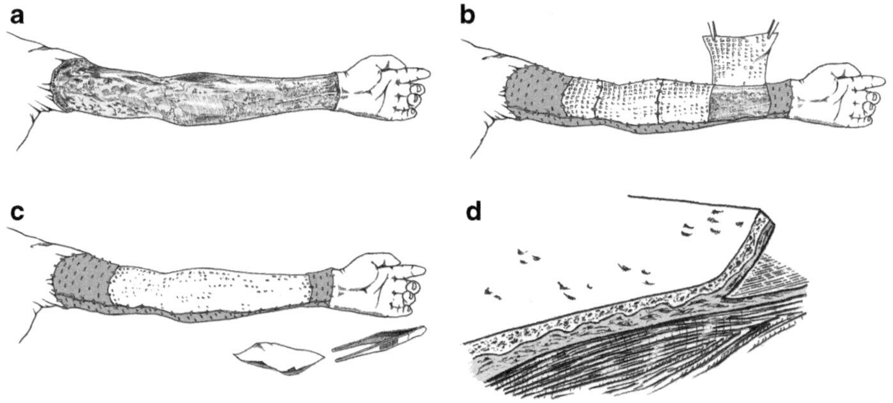

Fig. 3.1 One cycle of in vivo cultivation of autologous skin grafts. (**a**) The burned extremity is excised to the dermal or deep fascial layer. (**b**) Meek microskin grafts are meticulously applied to the freshly excised wound bed. (**c**) Approximately 10 days later, dressings are removed, full epithelialization of the interstices in the Meek grafts is achieved, and cultivation of autologous skin grafts is accomplished. (**d**). The newly cultivated autologous skin can be harvested with an electric dermatome

This cultivation cycle can be repeated as necessary to meet demands.

The newly cultivated autologous skin grafts can be used in various grafting techniques, such as microskin grafting, intermingled autologous and allogeneic skin grafting, Meek microskin grafting, and postage-stamp skin grafting.

The preferred sites for cultivation are the excised flexor surfaces in the anterior antebrachial or brachial region, as well as the posterior crural region. These sites are chosen due to their robust vascular supply to the underlying musculature, facilitating rapid growth of the transplanted Meek microskin grafts, which progress to effective coverage of the wound surface and formation of a relatively large whole piece of autologous skin. If available, alternative sites are relatively large excised wounds with preserved dermal viability.

[Typical Case]

The patient, a 51 years old man, sustained flame burns all over the body from an explosion of a tanker truck. Two hours after the injury, he arrived at a local hospital, where he received a tracheotomy, fluid resuscitation, escharotomies of the extremities and thorax, and anti-infection therapy. On the same day, he developed renal failure and anuria, for which hemodialysis was administered. On the third day post-injury, the director of our center was requested to lead the treatment team for the patient at the local hospital.

Admission diagnoses: (1) Burn size, 99.5% TBSA; burn depth, third-degree; (2) inhalation injury with tracheotomy; (3) renal failure.

Physical examination by burn specialist: A limited area of unaffected skin was identified in the patient's waist and bilateral axillae, covering approximately 0.5% TBSA. The rest of the skin, including the scalp and perineal skin, exhibited burn injuries characterized by a leathery appearance, evident thrombosed vessels, and loss of sensation.

First round of in vivo cultivation of autologous skin grafts: On the sixth day post-injury, excision of both upper and left lower extremities, autologous skin harvesting from the lower back and bilateral axillae, Meek grafting and allogeneic skin grafting were performed. About 140 cm^2 of split-thickness autologous skin was harvested from the lower back and bilateral axillae using an electric dermatome and fabricated into 1:4 Meek grafts, which were all grafted to the wounds on the flexor side of both upper excised extremities ("the cultivation sites"). On the tenth day post-grafting, epithelialization grew into the space among skin islands in the Meek grafts and fused to achieve a full coverage of the wound.

Application of cultivated skin grafts from the first round of cultivation and the process of the second round of cultivation: On the 23rd day post-injury (the 17th day after the initiation of the first round of autologous skin cultivation), the abdomen and both thighs were excised and grafted with prefabricated large sheets of postage-stamp skin allo- and autografts (prefabricated large graft sheet, PLGS) (see Sect. 3.2.1); skin grafts were harvested from the cultivation sites on both upper extremities; Meek grafting to repair the cultivation sites was again performed. Specifically, about 560cm^2 of the newly constructed autologous skin was harvested with an electric dermatome, among which 140cm^2 was fabricated into 1:4 Meek grafts and back-transplanted to the same cultivation sites on both upper extremities. The other 420 cm^2 was cut into 0.7 cm × 0.7 cm postage-stamp skin pieces using a quick cutting machine (Kexing Bio, Jiangxi, China) and together with 0.7 cm × 0.7 cm postage-stamp skin allografts fabricated into a PLGS for later use. The lower abdomen and both thigh roots were excised to the deep fascial layer and after complete hemostasis received PLGSs. Ten days later, all skin grafts on the recipient sites of the abdomen and both thighs survived, and full coverage of the wound of the cultivation sites was also obtained (see Fig. 3.2).

Application of cultivated skin grafts from second round of cultivation and the process of the third round of cultivation: On the 39th day post-injury, skin graft harvesting and Meek grafting for the same cultivation sites on both upper extremities were repeated, and both lower extremities received excision and PLGSs. To be specific, about 550 cm^2 of the newly constructed autologous skin was harvested and 140 cm^2 was fabricated into 1:4 Meek grafts and back-transplanted to the same cultivation sites. The rest was cut into 0.7 cm × 0.7 cm postage-stamp skin pieces and, together with 0.7 cm × 0.7 cm postage-stamp skin allografts, fabricated into PLGSs which were later grafted to both lower extremities after proper excision and complete hemostasis. All skin grafts on the recipient sites in both lower extremities survived. Full coverage of the wound of the cultivation sites was also obtained on the tenth day post-grafting.

Patient outcome: The 35-day management led by the director was critical and achieved successful results. The subsequent course of treatment was accomplished by the local staff. The patient was eventually discharged upon good recovery.

[Discussion]

The process of managing extensive burns is like a tug of war between wound repair and wound deterioration, as well as between complication prevention and complication outburst. If complications are well controlled, advances of wound repair would outpace complication development and bring about a final successful treatment. On the contrary, if complications outrace wound repair, the treatment would fail. The management of superficial wounds just needs to wait for enough time to achieve complete healing after dressing changes, while that of deeper wounds races against

Fig. 3.2 The strategy of in vivo cultivation of autologous skin grafts to treat a patient with 99.5% TBSA burns. (**a**) General view of the patient on the sixth day post-injury. (**b**) Excision was performed for the left upper extremity. (**c**) 1:4 Meek autografts were grafted to its flexor surface for in vivo cultivation. (**d**) The newly cultivated autologous skin on the tenth day post-grafting B, C, D: the first round of cultivation. (**e**) Wound surface of the cultivation site on the left upper extremity after harvesting. (**f**) Grafts harvested from the cultivation site. (**g**) 1:4 Meek autografts were back-grafted to the cultivation site for the second round of cultivation. (**h**) The newly cultivated autologous skin from the second round of cultivation on the tenth day post-grafting E, G, H: the second round of cultivation. (**i**) Excision was performed for the lower abdomen and roots of both lower extremities. (**j**) Prefabricated large sheets of postage-stamp skin allo- and autografts (prefabricated large graft sheet, or PLGS) were applied to the excised area. (**k**) Condition of the lower abdomen and roots of both lower extremities on the third day post-operation. (**l**) Condition of the lower abdomen and roots of both lower extremities on the tenth day post-operation

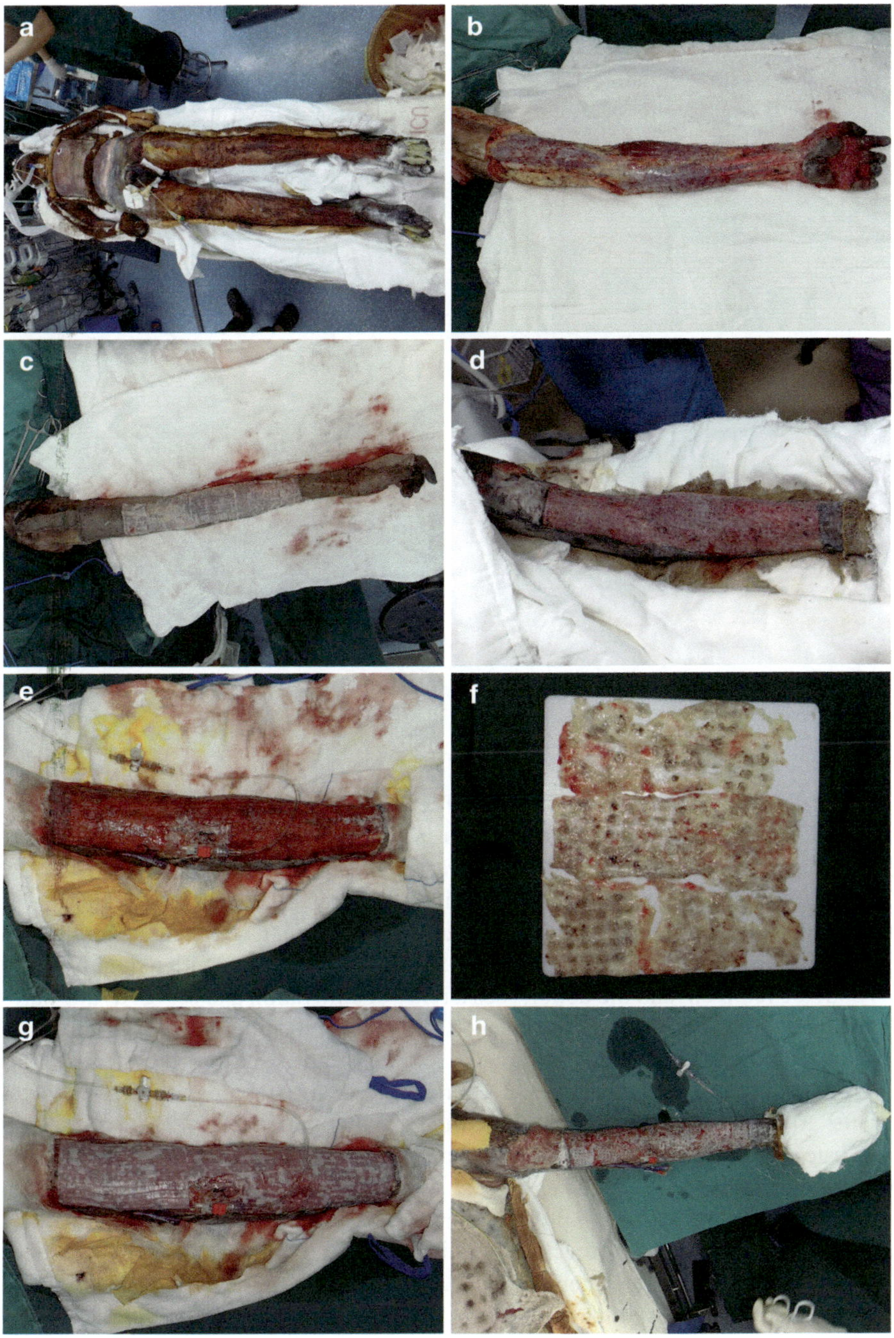

Fig. 3.2 (continued)

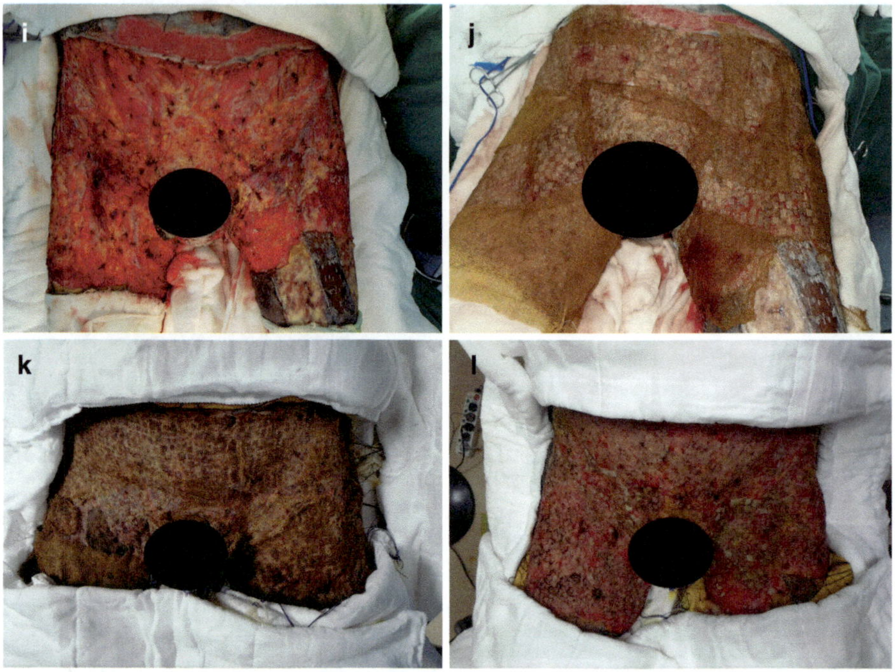

Fig. 3.2 (continued)

time since skin grafting is required [1]. Therefore, for the repair of extensive burn wounds, a sufficient source of autologous skin is the key to shorten the time for wound repair and ensure the success of treatment [6].

Technically facilitated by Meek grafting, the strategy of in vivo cultivation of autologous skin grafts we propose aims to grow sufficient, serviceable autologous skin grafts from the scarce surviving skin. The cultivation site, with a dual function as both the recipient and the donor, sees a relay of cultivation and serves as an "autograft bank" that accommodates repeated harvesting, thereby addressing the challenge of autograft paucity. The novelty of the strategy is that the treatment is navigated through the conventional course of "passive repair with limited autografts" to the new mode of "active cultivation of autografts" [7].

Histopathological analysis showed that, though the thickness of the epidermal layer in the two sections of the cultivated skin and the intact skin had no significant difference, the cultivated skin presented more collagen in the dermis than the intact skin, reflecting its better protective function [8]. In addition, immunofluorescence staining revealed a higher intensity of Ki-67 expression in the cultivated skin, suggesting the enhanced stemness and increased proliferative activities in the epidermal cells, which give rise to their fast adherence to, and expansive regeneration on,

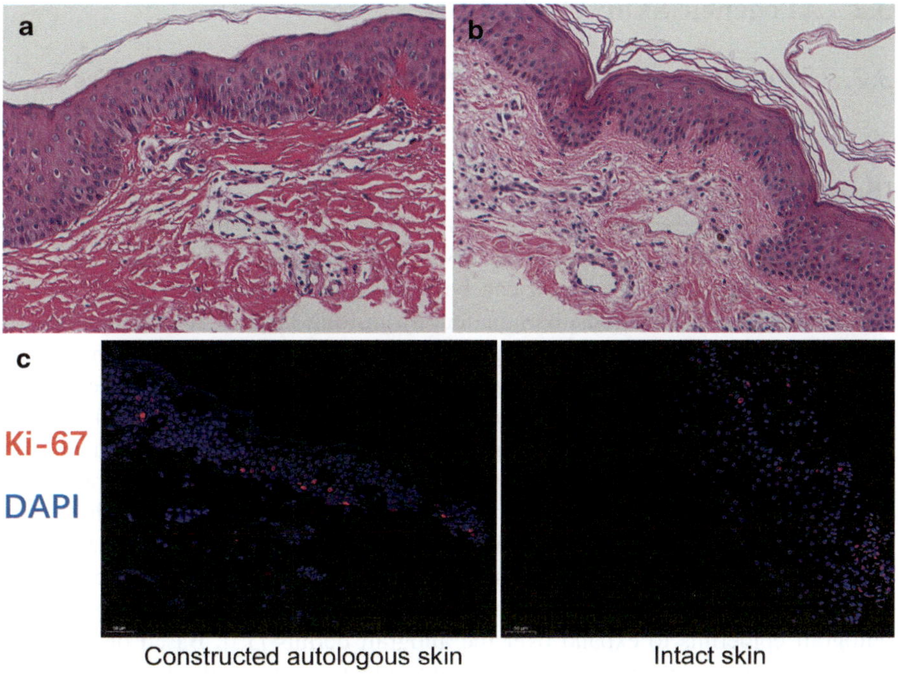

Fig. 3.3 Pathological comparison between the constructed autologous skin and the intact skin. (**a**) HE staining of the cultivated autologous skin from the first round. (**b**) HE staining of the intact skin from the same patient. (**c**) Representative immunofluorescence images of Ki-67 (red) staining and DAPI (blue) for the cultivated autologous skin and intact skin

the basal layer (Fig. 3.3) [9]. These findings demonstrate the rather satisfactory performance of the newly constructed autologous skin in wound repair.

The choice of the excised flexor surfaces in the anterior antebrachial or brachial region, or the posterior crural region, as the cultivation sites is based on their anatomical structure and our clinical experience. In our experience, these muscle-rich areas can deliver the most stable survival and regenerative expansion of the Meek grafts. Notably, an excised second-degree burn wound with residual dermis can facilitate a more stable Meek grafting and faster fusion of the grafts [10]. Therefore, if available, they are a better choice for the in vivo cultivation of autologous skin than those without residual dermis. The time to achieve fusion among the skin islands of the Meek grafts with different expansion ratios can vary greatly. It requires approximately 7 days for grafts with a 1:3 expansion ratio to achieve fusion, 10 days for a 1:4 ratio, and around 14 days for a 1:6 ratio [1]. We all know that time is of the essence when saving the lives of burn patients, and in most cases, we would like to choose Meek grafts with a 1:4 expansion ratio due to its balanced performance considering both the expansion ratio and fusion time.

3.2 Allogeneic Skin: Clinical Use

3.2.1 Prefabricated Large Graft Sheet (PLGS) for Extensive Burn Wounds

[Background]
Achieving adequate coverage for extensive deep burns has been a long-standing challenge since autografts would be severely insufficient in such cases [11]. In efforts to tackle the challenge, it can be noted that Jackson D, in 1954, made a breakthrough when he cured a burn patient by grafting strips of auto- and allografts alternately. This introduced intermingled grafting into the field of burn management [12]. However, with this approach, sufficient autografts are required, and extensive wounds could not be fully covered at one sitting. Then, in 1961, a modification to this technique was made—Tsi-Siang S and his colleagues placed alternatively laid postage-stamp auto- and allografts (1.0 cm × 1.0 cm) where the autograft strips should be placed in Jackson's method and leave the allograft strips where they should be [13]. With this modification, the limited autograft could be utilized more efficiently [14]. Compared with the strip pattern, the allograft rejection was weaker with the bricklaying style, where the allograft epidermis separated, allowing the autograft epidermis to expand over the allograft dermis [15]. Based on this, Xia Zhaofan et al. made a further improvement, placing auto- and allografts alternatively where the allograft strips were laid in Tsi-Siang S′ method. This enhanced method yielded improved outcomes [16].

The advantage of the bricklaying pattern is that the allografts that were deployed to improve autograft utilization efficiency would be vascularized to facilitate effective wound coverage. Such coverage minimizes wound exposure and desiccation, preventing infections, and limiting exudation and energy consumption. However, both bricklaying methods involve a piece-by-piece grafting process that is labor-intensive and time-consuming, which means an inappropriately prolonged general anesthesia for the patients, and thus render the methods inapplicable in real extensive burn care settings.

This issue can be effectively addressed by our new approach presented in this section [17]. The key to our approach is to prefabricate large sheets of uniformly arranged composite skin grafts, which can then be directly and neatly applied to the prepared wound bed. All the grafts are placed in a bricklaying pattern on a sterile stainless-steel plate, sprayed with Meek adhesive, and glued to a large piece of single gauze that serves as a carrier. The prefabrication should be completed before wound preparation is accomplished. Once careful excision, thorough debridement, and adequate hemostasis are achieved, the prefabricated large graft sheet (PLGS) can be applied. With the PLGS approach, the intraoperative grafting time significantly shortens from several hours in the conventional piecemeal way to only several minutes.

[Protocol]

Evaluation on patient condition and determination on the auto- to allograft ratio

Preoperatively, a careful size measurement of the autologous donor skin (A, cm^2) and the target wound (B, cm^2) is conducted. The ratio of auto- to allograft is presented as 1:N. N is the value that was first calculated with (B/A-1) and subsequently rounded to the nearest integer. Figure 3.4 shows the validated optimal layouts for different N values.

Construction of the PLGS

Two hours before the operation, a proper amount of cryopreserved viable allogeneic skin is obtained and thoroughly washed with saline. Then a skin graft cutting machine (Kexing Bio, Jiangxi, China) is deployed to cut the rinsed skin into small squares measuring 0.7 cm × 0.7 cm. All the small skin squares are arranged in advance on a sterilized and flat surface, for example, the back of a large surgical tray, and the positions for autografts are reserved in accordance with the optimal layout for the previously determined auto- to allograft ratio. Be careful to make sure that the epidermis side of all small grafts faces upward (Fig. 3.5a). Upon the completion of the placement of all the allografts, anesthesia of the patient is initiated. During the operation, an electric dermatome is used to harvest a split-thickness autologous graft (0.3 mm thick). After removal of blood and hair residues with saline, the autografts are also cut into small squares measuring 0.7 cm × 0.7 cm and then placed in the reserved positions on the back surface of the plate (Fig. 3.5b).

When the placement step is finalized, the plate is slightly tilted to drain residual saline. Then an even spray of MEEK Adhesive (Humeca, Borne, The Netherlands) to the arranged surface from roughly 25 cm away is performed, and it generally will form an even, tacky layer in 5 min. This tacky surface then receives a large piece of single gauze (Haomei, Xinxiang, China). To secure attachment, the gauze should be carefully pressed, and the product let stand for another 5 min and then lifted in a short-edge flip manner (Fig. 3.6). Redundant gauze can be trimmed. The lifted sheet is then relocated in a saline-containing tray. This process should be completed before wound preparation ends.

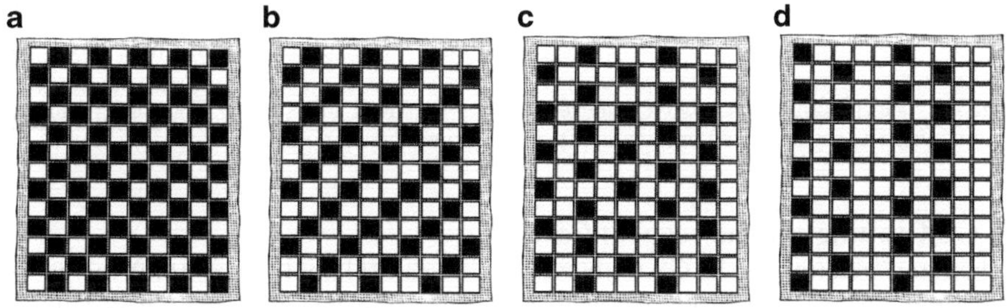

Fig. 3.4 Optimal layouts for different auto- to allograft ratios (1: N). (**a**). N = 1. (**b**) N = 2. (**c**) N = 3. (**d**) N = 4. Black, postage-stamp autografts; white, postage-stamp allografts. It should be noted that all postage-stamp grafts are positioned with an inter-graft distance of 0.1–0.2 mm

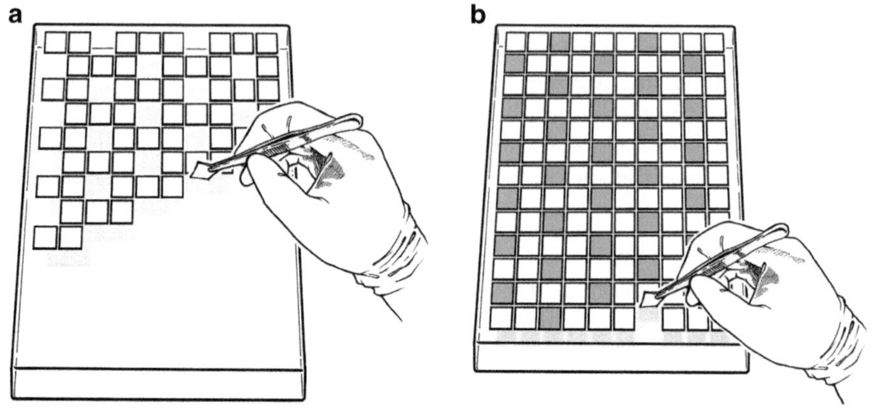

Fig. 3.5 Before the operation starts, postage-stamp allografts are placed according to the chosen layout for the calculated N value (**a**). During the operation, postage-stamp autografts are put into the reserved positions (**b**). All grafts are spaced 0.1–0.2 mm apart

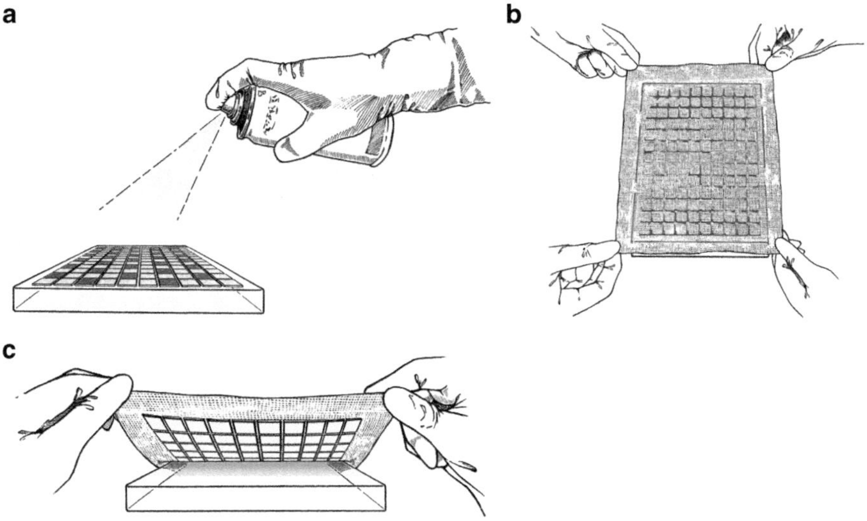

Fig. 3.6 The epidermal side receives an even spray of the Meek adhesive (**a**). The carrier gauze is applied (**b**). The prefabricated product is lifted by flipping the short edge (**c**)

PLGS Grafting and Subsequent Care

When transplanting the PLGS to the wound, be careful not to overstretch the gauze since the take rate might be undermined. After transplantation, the grafted site is dressed with a layer of fine gauze impregnated with silver sulfadiazine. Then layers of coarse gauze are used for enhanced compression and wrapping. Three days post-operatively, the outer dressings can be opened to allow routine inspection of the grafted site. The absence of undesirable conditions such as excess exudation and infections indicates that the inner carrier gauze can be retained for the following 2 to 3 weeks, during which the outer dressings should be renewed every other day. During dressing renewals, signs of excess exudation indicate that the retained carrier gauze should be removed and proper antibiotics given. Shedding of the postage-stamp grafts is often inevitable. For small-size wound exposures, conservative treatment typically works, while for larger ones, additional grafting of small autograft pieces is often needed. Generally, in postoperative care, anti-rejection medications and immunosuppressants are not necessary.

Indications

This approach is aptly suited for large-size excised wounds. The conventional method is not suited for cases requiring grafting on the entire posterior trunk, or the entire upper or lower extremity, due to the extended duration (often several hours) involved in the piece-by-piece and in situ positioning. For these cases, the proposed approach proves advantageous, as it substantially reduces the time taken to cover the target area to a mere few minutes.

[Typical Case]

A 44-year-old woman sustained extensive flame burns in a gas cylinder explosion. She was admitted to our center 6 h post-injury and diagnosed with burns covering 85%TBSA (third-degree, 53%TBSA), along with inhalation injuries. After admission, she received fluid resuscitation, tracheotomy, mechanical ventilation, debridement, dressing change, and burn intensive care. On the fifth day post-admission, the patient was in a stable condition and received tangential excision, escharectomy and coverage by allografts on the left lower extremity. Twelve days later (17 days post-burn), the left lower extremity was rid of the allografts, debrided, and then received PLGS grafting. The autologous donor skin area was measured to be 460 cm^2 and that of the graft sites was 2400 cm^2. As the patient voluntarily participated in our study to evaluate the presented approach, 100 cm^2 out of the 2400 cm^2 wound was selected to receive in situ piece-by-piece grafting. Therefore, a 2300 cm^2 PLGS was constructed, in accordance with the optimal layout for 1:4. The procedure of ex situ positioning took 70 min. In contrast, the in situ piece-by-piece positioning on the selected area was finished by two surgeons in 9 min, while the PLGS transplantation for the remaining 2300 cm^2 took merely 8 minutes.

Subsequent to the operation, a routine of dressing changes was performed every other day. On the 17th day post-grafting (34 days post-burn), the carrier gauze of the PLGS was removed. The take rate was approximately 90%. By the 30th day post-grafting (47 days post-burn), it was observed that the allograft epidermis separated and the autograft epidermis grew and covered the allograft dermis. A complete wound closure was finally achieved, and the patient was discharged with satisfactory recovery.

Eleven months later, a follow-up visit revealed a smooth and pliable surface of the PLGS-grafted area, with no noticeable hypertrophic scars or contracture. And the knee joint functions satisfactorily in activities, extension, and flexion (Fig. 3.7).

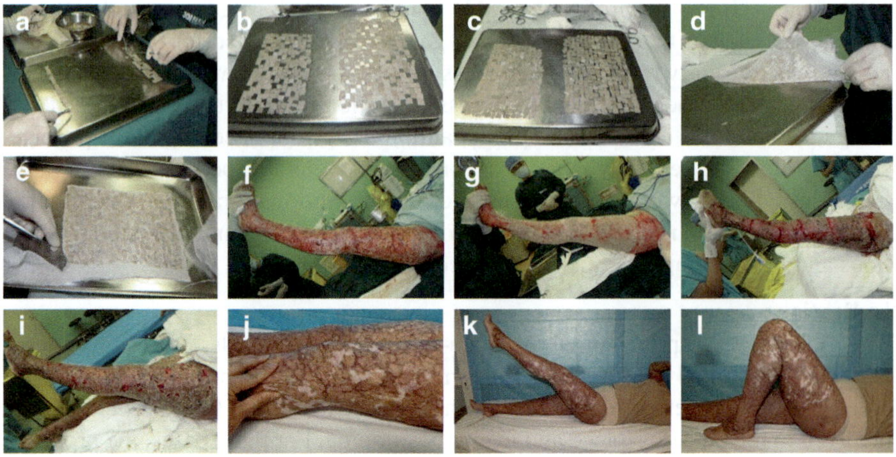

Fig. 3.7 R = 2. Postage-stamp allografts were carefully positioned (**a**, **b**). Postage-stamp autografts filled in the reserved places (**c**). The adhesive was sprayed, the carrier gauze applied, the PLGS lifted and relocated in a saline-containing tray (**d**, **e**). The left lower extremity received excision (**f**) and PLGS grafting (**g**). On the 17th day post-grafting, the carrier gauze was removed (**h**). The grafted area healed 30 days post-grafting (**i**). Follow-up 11 months later revealed satisfactory results (**j**, **k**, **l**)

[Discussion]

Burn professionals' priorities in treating extensive deep burns have always been to remove necrotic tissue and to achieve effective wound coverage in a timely manner. The two goals are set to ensure reduced patient mortality by preventing severe complications such as infections, tissue lysis, and undue wound exposure [18]. To date, for the permanent coverage of deep wounds, autografting remains the optimal choice. Since autografts are at a premium in extensive burn cases, it is ideal to maximize their utilization efficiency. In various efforts to achieve this, the Jackson's method, the in situ piece-by-piece grafting method, and the sandwich grafting approach represent the previous endeavors to deploy allografts in supporting autografting.

Compared with methods involving xenografts, these endeavors augment autograft use while ensuring effective coverage and take rate. This can be attributed to the vascularization of the allografts. Effective wound coverage protects the wound from desiccation, exudation, and infections. Studies revealed that 7 days after intermingled grafting in a bricklaying manner, a rejection response would occur, causing allografts' epidermal cell necrosis. Concurrently, the autografts' epithelial layer grows and gradually creeps over the dermal layer of the allografts. Or it can be said that the allografts' dermal layer gradually sandwiches the autografts' epithelial layer and the underlying connective tissue layer together (3). In animal models, it has been demonstrated that about 28 days after intermingled grafting in a bricklaying manner, a complete fusion of the autografts' epidermis, or a full wound coverage, could be observed (6). It is recommended that the size of the postage-stamp graft should be maintained above 0.09 cm^2 but limited as much as possible. The spacing between the grafts should be limited within 1.0 cm. The two recommendations help minimize potential wound exposure by aligning the paces between autograft epidermal expansion and the allograft epidermal exfoliation. Xia Zhaofan et al. reported successful outcomes with intermingled grafting in wound repair, with follow-ups over 1–2 years showing smooth and pliable resurfaced skin with mild scars [16].

Currently, the laborious process of graft positioning has not been automated yet and continues to rely on manual and piece-by-piece placement. This results in a prolonged operative time and increases the associated operative risks. From our experience, a full dorsal burn in an adult patient requires approximately 4 h to receive all the postage-stamp grafts piece-by-piece, even when four surgeons work simultaneously. This extends the anesthesia slot and lengthens wound exposure, which would exacerbate desiccation in viable tissue. This may extend injury depth and increase the risk of infections, which can be particularly detrimental in extensive deep burn cases. Meanwhile, prolonged operative time also compromises autograft vitality. Therefore, an effective and optimized strategy to minimize operative time for intermingled grafting would be valuable.

Our approach introduces the construction of PLGS, which significantly boosts efficiency and is easy to replicate. Initially tested on small wounds measuring approximately 1600 cm^2, the technique demonstrated stable and favorable performance. Further, it has been applied to large-size excised wounds, with the largest area covered with PLGS reaching 4300 cm^2.

The layouts for PLGS construction can differ significantly for different auto- to allograft ratios (1:N). This section just presents several optimal layouts that can minimize the largest distance between autografts, which facilitates optimal autograft fusion and speeds coverage. With the determination of the N value, it is easy for surgeons to follow the corresponding layout to position the postage-stamp grafts. This makes the procedure streamlined with enhanced efficiency and uniformity.

A proper distance should be maintained when spraying the adhesive onto the skin surface. The distance should be neither too short nor too long so as to avoid graft displacement and impaired spray efficiency. From our experience, a distance of 25 cm is advised. To ensure strong adhesion of all grafts to the carrier gauze, a proper amount of spray is advised to facilitate the formation of a tacky glue layer, but excessive glue should also be avoided to prevent occlusion of the holes of the gauze and undermining of drainage. And theoretically, with this approach, superior healing results can be expected with a higher auto- to allo-graft ratio. In our work, satisfactory outcomes have been achieved with an auto- to allo-graft ratio of 1:4. Further studies for smaller ratios can be anticipated.

It should be mentioned that there are some other widely utilized approaches to augment the use of the limited autografts. For instance, Akita S et al. reported that cultured epithelial autografts (CEA) combined with 1:6 mesh grafting yielded results comparable to those obtained with conventional 1:3 meshes [19]. Both this approach and ours utilize physiological dressings to achieve full coverage for the wound. However, a key distinction between the two is that 3 to 4 weeks are required to prepare the cultures in the CEA method, whereas that time can be saved with our method since allografts are readily available [20]. This makes our method well-suited to early surgical interventions for large-size deep wounds.

[Conclusion]
To summarize, the proposed approach emphasizes the change from in situ positioning of postage-stamp autografts following wound preparation to ex situ prefabrication of a large graft sheet simultaneous with the wound preparation. This change is beneficial to intermingled grafting with postage-stamp skin grafts; it is an excellent method per se, but impractical in treating extensive deep burns. With the proposed approach, it is now feasible. The approach provides a smart complement to the existing treatment system for extensive deep burns.

3.2.2 Fresh Allogenic Scalp for Pediatric Burn Wounds

Background
Pediatric burn management, though with its specific features, also demands early effective coverage after wound excision. The issue of limited available autologous skin has prompted burn professionals to seek substitutes for effective coverage. Among all possible alternatives, allografts serve as the secondary choice to autograft for coverage and are typically categorized into three types: fresh allograft, cryopreserved allograft, and glycerol-preserved allograft. The utilization of allografts was first proposed by Reverdin in 1869 [21], and in the same year, Girdner for the first time employed cadaveric skin for large burn wound coverage [22]. At that time, the allogeneic skin was all fresh and could not be preserved for extended periods. In 1966, Cochrane reported the successful application of cryopreserved allografts in wound management. In 1973, our center established a skin tissue bank and preserved skin tissue at 4 °C, −20 °C, and −80 °C as well as −195.8 °C in liquid nitrogen. Preservation at 4 °C led to rapid viability decline, while storage at −20 °C, −80 °C, and −195.8 °C allowed for long-term preservation, with graft viability remaining acceptable even after 5 years, ensuring graft availability for burn treatment. The development of glycerol-preserved allografts in Holland in 1984 introduced advantages such as enhanced handling and storage convenience, viral inhibition by glycerol, lower costs, and reduced antigenicity compared to cryopreserved allografts. However, concerns persist regarding the efficacy of glycerol in eliminating hepatitis viruses and HIV. While glycerolization maintains anatomical structure and strength, it diminishes tissue vitality and anti-infective properties.

Recent stringent regulations governing organ transplantation have restricted access to allogeneic (primarily cadaveric) skin, presenting a new hurdle in burn care. In response, the author proposes utilizing fresh scalp tissue from pediatric patients' relatives for burn wound treatment, a method successfully employed over the past decade at our institution for large burns in pediatric patients. This approach offers a dependable source of donor skin and has yielded favorable outcomes.

Indications

1. Pediatric burn wounds with a size of 30% TBSA or greater in the early stage post-burn
2. Pediatric burn wounds complicated by infection
3. Willingness of the donor relative to donating skin and fulfillment of the inclusion criteria outlined in the "Inclusion criteria for scalp donors" section

Contradictions

1. Patient's medical condition precludes surgical intervention.
2. Lack of willingness from the relative to donate skin grafts.

Pre-operative arrangements

1. **Routine preoperative preparation**

   The pediatric patients, aged 12 years or younger with large burns, are given standard preoperative measures including anti-shock and anti-infection fluid administration, organ protection, nutritional support, and blood transfusion as needed. The first operation is typically scheduled between the third and fifth day post-burn, with priority given to extremities before the trunk. Before operation, a deep intravenous line is established, arterial pressure monitoring is performed, hypoproteinemia is corrected to maintain Hb $\geq$ 100 g/L, and obvious abnormalities in coagulation and cardiopulmonary function are corrected. The patient's condition is carefully assessed and the operation area determined. Generally, the size of the wounds to be excised in a single operation should not exceed 30% TBSA, and it would be favorable to complete the operation within a 3-hour timeframe. Preoperative team communication, thorough anesthesia evaluation, adequate transfusion preparation, and ensuring optimal operating room conditions, particularly warming up the room temperature, are integral components of the preoperative protocol.

2. **Determining operation size and allogeneic scalp skin requirement**

   The body surface area (BSA) of the patient is calculated with the *Stevenson formula*:

   $$BSA\left(\mathrm{m}^2\right) = 0.0061 \times \text{height}\left(\mathrm{cm}\right) + 0.0128 \times \text{body weight}\left(\mathrm{kg}\right) - 0.1529.$$

   For children aged 1, 2, and 7 years, the calculated BSA values are approximately 0.45m^2 (10 kg in weight), 0.58m^2 (13 kg in weight), and 0.9m^2 (25 kg in weight), respectively. The proportions of different body parts to BSA in children differ from that in adults. For instance, in a 1-year-old child, a unilateral trunk, upper extremity, and lower extremity represent approximately 16%, 9.5%, and 15% TBSA, with absolute sizes of 720 cm^2, 428 cm^2, and 664 cm^2, respectively (see Table 3.1). On average, the size of donor scalp skin from adults measured around 560 ± 60 cm^2 based on a cohort study of 94 cases. Given this data, it can be estimated that adult donor scalp skin can cover approximately 78%, 100%, and 84% of wounds on a unilateral trunk, unilateral upper extremity, and unilateral lower extremity, respectively. This efficiency in coverage underscores the practicality and effectiveness of utilizing adult donor scalp skin for pediatric burn wound management.

Table 3.1 Surface area of unilateral trunk, unilateral upper and lower extremities of children of different ages and different weights calculated with the *Stevenson formula*

Age	Body weight (kg)	Body surface area (m^2)	Unilateral trunk (cm^2)	Unilateral upper extremity (cm^2)	Unilateral lower extremity (cm^2)
4 months	6	0.30	495	285	405
1-year-old	10	0.45	720	428	664
2-year-old	13	0.58	899	551	928
7-year–old	25	0.90	1296	855	1733
12-year–old	40	1.30	1833	1261	2678

In the scenario where both an upper extremity and a lower extremity of a 1-year-old burn patient require coverage with fresh allogeneic scalp, totaling approximately 1092cm^2, a maximum of two adult donors would satisfy the need; for a 2-year-old, 1479 cm^2, three adult donors; for a 7-year-old, 2588 cm^2, five adult donors are needed. Practically, with efforts to utilize autografts wherever possible, the actual demand for allogeneic scalp will be less.

3. **Optimizing the utilization of the fresh allogeneic scalp**

   For cases with wound sepsis that require grafting, large pieces of fresh allogeneic scalp can be directly applied to the excised wounds. This approach serves to expedite surgical procedures and protect the wound surface.

   For cases with burn size ≥90% TBSA, fresh allogeneic scalp can be employed to cover the wounds that are left exposed after Meek autografting of other major wounds and await either autografting or intermingled transplantation of auto- and allografts in future procedures.

   For other cases, fresh allogeneic scalp, in conjunction with autologous skin, can be fashioned into postage-stamp skin grafts with side lengths ranging from 1 to 1.5 cm. These smaller grafts can be mixed in different ratios to effectively cover the wounds.

The Inclusion Criteria of Scalp Donors and Their Pre-op Preparations

A stringent set of inclusion criteria is implemented to safeguard the donor's recovery process and minimize risks for the recipient.

Inclusion criteria for scalp donors:

1. Age between 18 and 60 years
2. Demonstrates good or excellent nutritional status and a favorable health record
3. Must be a parent or relative of the child
4. Voluntarily participates and provides informed consent

Exclusion criteria for donor candidates:

1. Presence of severe underlying conditions like diabetes, coronary heart disease, or chronic pulmonary disorders
2. Women who are pregnant or breastfeeding

3. History of psoriasis, folliculitis, or alopecia on the scalp
4. Positive test results for syphilis, hepatitis B, hepatitis C, or HIV
5. Diagnosis of cervical spondylosis or limited neck mobility

Preoperative preparations:

Prior to surgery, a comprehensive medical history of the donor is obtained, and a thorough physical examination is conducted with special emphasis on neck mobility. Standard preoperative tests, including complete blood count (CBC), blood typing, liver and renal function assessments, coagulation studies, screening for HIV, hepatitis A, B, C, and TORCH infections, urinalysis, stool analysis, electrocardiogram (ECG), and chest X-rays, are performed. Additionally, donors of advanced age undergo echocardiography to evaluate cardiac function.

Perioperative protocol

It is recommended that the surgery for scalp donors be performed simultaneously with or prior to that of the recipient child, so as to permit a seamless transplantation process, eliminate delays in waiting for the scalp to be prepared, reduce operative risks, and enhance overall efficiency.

1. **Harvesting and handling of fresh scalp skin from donor relatives**

   The donor undergoes general anesthesia for the procedure. Prior to skin harvest, a solution of epinephrine in normal saline (1 μg/ml, 800–1000 ml) is injected under the galea aponeurotica. Split-thickness scalp skin, containing dermal papillae, is then harvested using a Zimmer electric dermatome (thickness: 0.25–0.3 mm; size: 3% TBSA). The harvested skin is meticulously rinsed with normal saline three times to eliminate any blood and hair residues. Subsequently, the skin is either cut into postage-stamp skin grafts (side length: 1–1.5 cm) or perforated (diameter: 2–3 mm) to improve drainage post-application.

   The donor site is compressed with epinephrine-soaked gauze for hemostasis and then covered with fine-mesh gauze impregnated with Vaseline on which multiple layers of sterile gauze dressings are utilized to provide additional compression and secure wrapping.
2. **Wound preparation and grafting for the pediatric patient**

   General anesthesia is performed for the recipient patient. For extremity grafting, a tourniquet is employed at the root to contain blood flow to the surgical field. For trunk grafting, a proper amount of solution containing epinephrine (1 μg/ml in normal saline) is injected along the margin of the surgical field with a long needle to minimize operative blood loss. Tangential excision is performed to preserve as much viable dermal tissue as possible for deep second-degree burn wounds, while excision to healthy fat tissue or deeper fascia is performed for third-degree wounds. Ooze from small vessels is stopped with electrocautery, while larger vessels are ligated when encountered. Particular attention is paid to preventing excessive blood loss and the potential hemorrhagic shock during trunk operations, where tourniquets are not applicable. Upon the completion of wound preparation, i.e., debridement and hemostasis, the wound is temporarily covered with sterile gauze moistened with normal saline until grafting. An adequate amount of autologous skin from proper sites is obtained and made into postage-stamp skin grafts or Meek grafts for later use.

In accordance with the individualized treatment plan, the fresh allogeneic scalp skin grafts, either alone or along with the autologous skin grafts, are applied to the wounds. These grafts are further covered with layers of mesh gauze and secured with staples to prevent displacement. After this, a single layer of fine mesh gauze dressing impregnated with silver sulfadiazine and multiple layers of coarse mesh gauze dressings are used to compress and wrap the grafted site. For grafting procedures involving the knees and elbows, proper splints can be employed to restrict joint mobility.

Post-operation management

For the donor sites of the relative, the inner fine-mesh gauze impregnated with Vaseline can be retained, while the outer layers of sterile gauze dressings are typically removed between day 1 and 3 post-harvesting, depending on the level of exudation. Topical application of Baikerui® Disinfectant Spray (Shanghai Hi-tech Bioengineering Co Ltd., China), which contains the compounds lysostaphin and chlorhexidine acetate, or adf® 0.5% PVP-I Disinfectant Solution, followed by rhEGF, is performed three to four times daily and dried with a dryer. The donor sites are regularly inspected for recovery monitoring. Excessive exudation under the Vaseline gauze calls for immediate clearance. The Vaseline gauze can typically be removed between day 8 and 10 post-harvesting and may be kept longer for slower wound healing.

In caring for the pediatric patient, monitoring general condition and vital signs is routine, accompanied by regular tests such as CBC, coagulation studies, liver and renal function studies, electrolytes, B-type natriuretic peptide (BNP), and procalcitonin. Appropriate antibiotics are given based on the patient's symptoms, bacterial culture results, and response to different antibiotics. Vigorous nutritional support and an adequate supply of red cell suspension and plasma are given to maintain Hb $\geq$ 100 g/L and ALB $\geq$35 g/L.

For pediatric recipient sites, the outer dressings can be gently opened for the first time between days 5 and 7 to inspect the grafted wound, while the inner layer of mesh gauze is retained. Subsequently, dressings are changed every other day. A slow, gentle, and careful removal of the dressings and careful inspection of the allografts are crucial. Obvious exudation necessitates localized drainage and disinfection to maintain cleanliness and dryness. The use of disinfectant in a large dose should be avoided, and topical epidermal growth promoters such as rhEGF may be prescribed. During the second dressing change, the inner mesh gauze should be removed, after which disinfection and topical application of epidermal growth promoters are repeated. Adequate compression and wrapping during the first two dressing changes are necessary to prevent graft disruption. Two to three weeks postoperative, gradual exfoliation of the allografts occurs; partial coverage by the creeping neighboring autografts of the areas where the allografts exfoliated, healing of the underlying deep second-degree wounds, a residue of the allogeneic dermal components, or a complete exposure of the underlying granulation bed may be observed. At this time, additional grafting with either autologous skin or allogeneic scalp skin can be considered until complete healing is achieved. Upon complete healing, anti-scar treatment and functional training are begun.

Typical Cases
Case no. 1

The patient, a 7-year-old boy, sustained burns over his body due to a gas explosion. He received tracheotomy and anti-shock therapy at a local hospital and 2 days later was transferred to our center.

Admission diagnoses: 1. Burn size, 90% TBSA; burn depth, 85% third-degree, 5% deep second-degree; 2. severe inhalation injury; 3. wound sepsis; 4. electrolyte imbalance; 5. post-tracheotomy.

Specialized physical exams: The patient sustained burns with a total size of 90% TBSA (Fig. 3.8). Patches of unburned skin were found on the abdomen, buttocks, and both lower extremities. Significant edema was observed on the head and face, with the burn sites covered in eschar. The eyelids exhibited eversion due to edema, and the mouth, with pronounced swelling lips, resembled the mouth of a fish. The wounds on the posterior trunk were classified as third-degree burns, displaying a leathery appearance and signs of exfoliation. The anterior neck wounds shed eschar and exposed a pale base. Both upper extremities were covered in eschar, with acceptable blood supply, and had escharotomies performed to the deep fascia layer for pressure reduction. Both lower extremities were mostly pale, with a few areas being pink, and temperatures of his fingers and toes were acceptable.

Treatment course: Early excision and skin grafting were performed for the patient to achieve a gradual wound coverage. Excision was performed in the forms of tangential excision, excision to healthy fat tissue or deeper fascia, dependent on the burn area and depth. Skin grafting methods include Meek skin grafting, postage-stamp allo- and autografting, and back-grafting to the patient's donor sites. In total, fresh allogeneic scalp skin obtained from 14 harvesting procedures was made into postage-stamp grafts and grafted to the wound alone or together with autologous skins. Take the wounds on the patient's back, for instance. These wounds were maintained in an open and sterile condition until day 22 post-burn when excision, partly to the fat layer and partly to the deep fascia layer, was performed. Due to the unavailability of appropriate autograft donor sites, fresh allogeneic scalp skin from two harvesting procedures was made into postage-stamp skin grafts to cover the wound. These grafts were subsequently secured and bandaged. Dressing changes were conducted in accordance with the aforementioned postoperative management protocol. The allografts began to shed 1 week post-grafting. Eleven days after the first operation the second operation was performed where the wound was excised and grafted with both autologous skin and allogeneic scalp skin obtained from one harvesting procedure. Ten days later, most of the allografts shed. Thirteen days after the second operation, the third operation was performed with both autologous skin and allogeneic scalp skin obtained from one harvesting procedure. Eventually, the back wounds healed 70 days post-injury. The follow-up one and a half years later showed that the resurfaced back had acceptable pliability and mild scars (Fig. 3.9). Subsequently, surgical corrections to release the contracture of the eyelids, the neck,

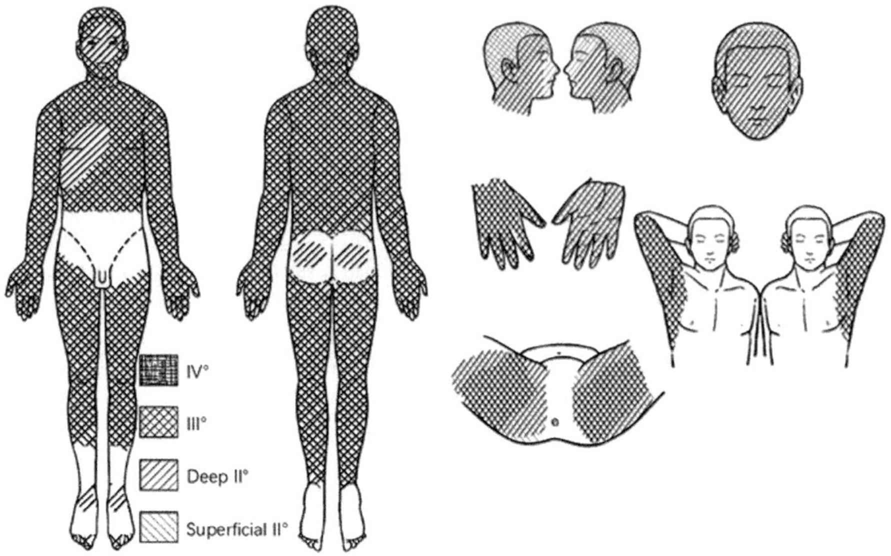

	Superficial II°	Deep II°	III°	IV°
Head		1	9	
Neck			3	
Trunk		2.5	19	
Upper Arms			7	
Lower arms			6	
Hands			5	
Buttocks		1	3	
Thighs			18	
Legs			9	
Feet		0.5	6	
Total		5%	85%	
Burn Size	90% TBSA			

Fig. 3.8 Burn profile of the 7-year-old patient

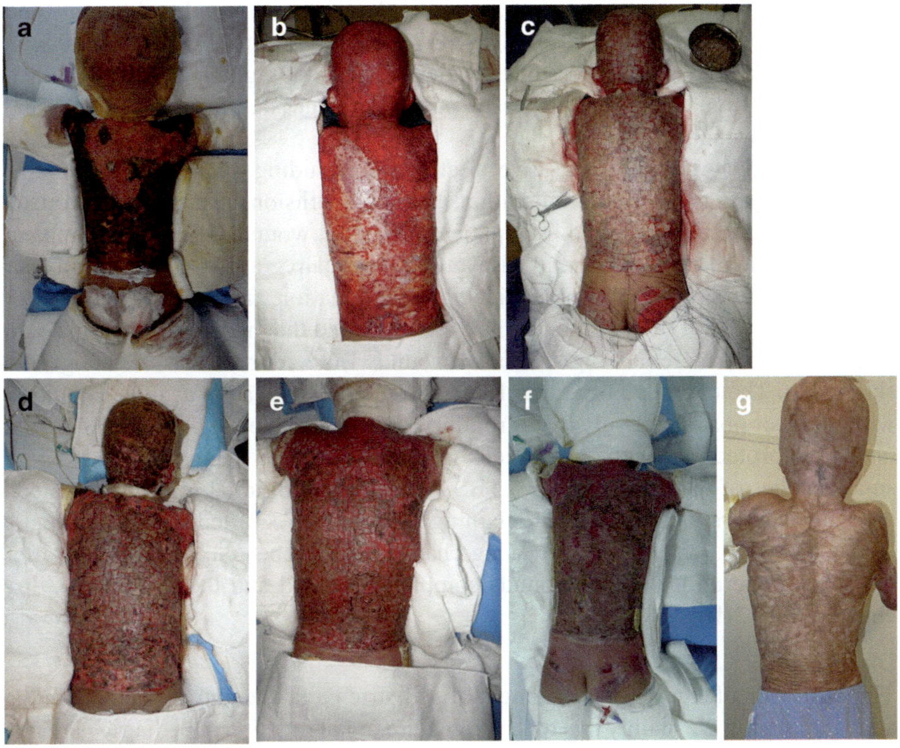

Fig. 3.9 The treatment course and prognosis of the burned back of the pediatric patient with a burn size of 90%TBSA. (**a**) Back wound surface 19 days post-burn. (**b**) Back wound surface prepared after excision during the first operation. (**c**) Fresh allogeneic scalp skin was made into postage-stamp grafts for wound coverage of the excised back. (**d**) Inspection of the wound surface 3 days post-operation. (**e**) Wound condition 46 days post-burn. (**f**). 70 days post-injury, the back basically healed. (**g**). Follow-up 1.5 years later showed satisfactory results

and both hands were performed. The patient eventually gained good recovery and was discharged.

Case no. 2

The patient, a 3-year-and-1-month-old boy, sustained multiple burns affecting the trunk, peritoneum, right upper extremity, and both lower extremities due to contact with hot liquid. He received wound dressing and anti-shock therapy at a local medical facility but, due to fever and decreased consciousness, was transferred to our center 1 week later.

Admission diagnoses: 1. Burn size, 24% TBSA (third-degree, 4%; deep second-degree, 20%); 2. wound sepsis; 3. hypoalbuminemia.

Specialized physical exams: The patient presented with a lucid mental state but exhibited signs of lethargy and reduced appetite. His urinary and bowel habits were normal. His vitals: body temp, 38.5 °C; pulse,124; RR, 20; BP, 88/74. His total burn size was 24% TBSA, involving the anterior trunk, peritoneum, right upper arm, and the anterior upper regions of both thighs. The wound base was mostly covered with necrotic tissue. The injured areas on the anterior trunk and right upper arm exhibited slight indentation, thick necrotic tissue adherence, and significant exudation and emitted a noticeable odor.

Treatment course: Conservative treatments, including anti-infective therapy, nutritional support, fluid administration, blood transfusion, and organ protection interventions, were performed. The patient presented wound sepsis, and complete coverage for his large-size wound with autologous scalp graft was unfeasible. Four days post-admission, his father provided a scalp donation, facilitating coverage for approximately 8% TBSA of the child's excised wound that had residual dermal and adipose tissue. The remaining shallower wounds were addressed with xenogeneic skin grafts. The operative time was 1.5 h, and the patient was in a stable condition without fever postoperatively. After routine dressing changes, most wounds healed under the protection of the allogeneic scalp skin and the xenogeneic skin, with small patches of wounds (about 3% TBSA) awaiting additional grafting. Nineteen days after the first operation, the remaining wounds were grafted with the patient's own scalp skin. Postoperative dressing changes were repeated, and 14 days after the second operation, all the wounds completely healed and the patient was discharged (Fig. 3.10).

Discussion

The greater challenges in the treatment of pediatric large-size burns than that in the adult population are mainly due to the premature organ function in pediatric patients, limited medication options, and rapid fluctuations in their condition [23]. However, a common principle shared between pediatric and adult burn care is the critical importance of achieving wound closure. Notably, good coverage material may significantly improve patient outcomes and prognosis.

In the treatment of pediatric large-size burns, fresh allogeneic scalp grafts offer several advantages:

- **Transitional coverage.** Fresh allogeneic scalp grafts can provide temporary coverage for wounds, preventing infections due to exposure, reducing exudation, ameliorating hypermetabolism, and thereby facilitating a smoother treatment course.
- **Better viability.** Compared with the glycerol-preserved and cryopreserved allogeneic skin and glycerol allogeneic skin, fresh allogeneic scalp grafts demonstrate superior vitality and higher survival rate within 7 days post-grafting (reaching up to 100% in the early stage), resembling the resilience of autologous skin.
- **Strong anti-infective properties.** These grafts provide effective protection for wounds, including infected ones. They provide a variety of growth factors that enhance the local microenvironment, promoting autograft survival and growth.
- **Extended donor site recovery window.** Fresh allogeneic scalp grafts can survive on the wound surface for approximately 2 weeks, creating an extended time window for donor site regeneration. Then after their exfoliation, the underlying

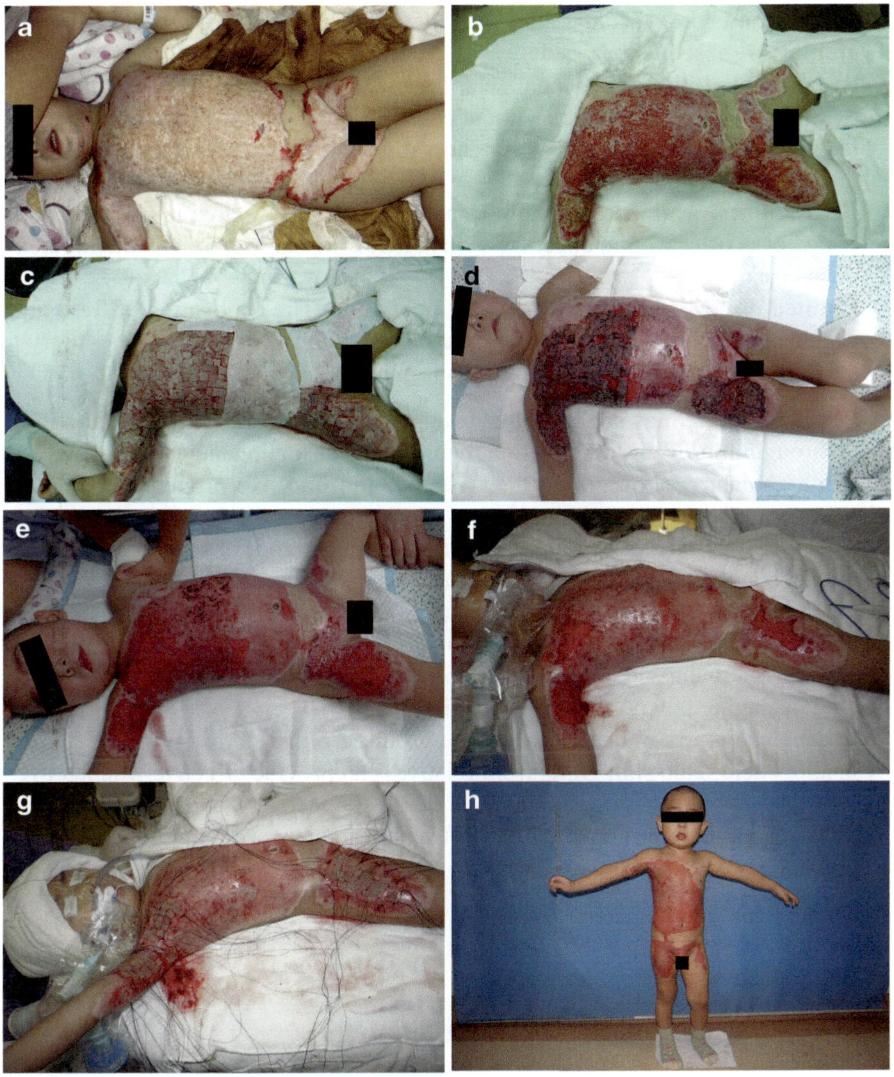

Fig. 3.10 The treatment course and outcome of the 3-year-old boy with severe scalds. (**a**) Wound status 1-week post-injury (upon admission to our center). (**b**) The wounds received debridement during the first operation. (**c**) The debrided wounds received grafting with allogeneic scalp skin grafts and xenogeneic skin grafts. (**d**) 7 days after the first operation. (**e**) 13 days after the first operation. (**f**) The residual wounds received debridement during the second operation. (**g**) The debrided wounds were grafted with the child's own scalp skin during the second operation. (**h**) Wound healing results upon discharge

granulation bed or residual allogeneic dermis would be well receptive to autografting in subsequent procedures.

- **Broad availability.** Allogeneic scalp skin can be sourced from healthy adult relatives of pediatric patients without concerns about crossmatching results. The fact that relatives often show willingness to donate with a sense of responsibility minimizes potential disputes.
- **Reduced financial burden.** With a smaller body surface area in children, adult scalp grafts offer wound coverage with higher efficiency, thereby reducing treatment costs.
- **Limited donor injury and favorable prognosis.** The application of fresh allogeneic scalp grafts parallels allogeneic blood or cell transfusions. The injury to the donor is limited, and the prognosis is generally good.

While the future may see increased availability of allogeneic skin for burn treatment through improved skin donation regulations, fresh allogeneic scalp grafts will remain a valuable option due to their vitality, anti-infective properties, and other aforementioned benefits [24].

Nonetheless, clinicians should stay alert to the occurrence of severe rejection and infectious complications, as fresh allogeneic scalp grafts can exhibit strong antigenicity and early rejection, typically occurring 2–3 weeks post-grafting. Though to date, no acute rejection event in the recipients has occurred in our experience, preoperative assessments and diligent postoperative monitoring are crucial to identifying and managing potential adverse reactions [25].

In conclusion, in regions where cutaneous allografts from cadavers are limited, fresh allogeneic scalp skin grafts from relatives can provide effective wound coverage and protection, extend the window for donor site recovery, and create conditions for subsequent autografting, serving as a feasible and powerful alternative for managing large burns in pediatric patients.

(Chuanan Shen, Huping Deng)

3.3 New Excision and Grafting Strategies

3.3.1 Extra-Large but Conservative Excision

[Background]

It is believed that in the management of extensive burns, the wound size to be excised in a single surgical session shall not exceed 30% TBSA. This guideline is based on the understanding that larger excisions can lead to significant blood loss, resulting in unstable patient conditions and heightened intraoperative risks. In our experience, the blood loss per 1% TBSA of the extremities excised averages between 80 and 100 ml [26], whereas that of the trunk or other areas where tourniquets cannot be employed will be substantially higher. Estimation can be made that an excision size exceeding 30% at one sitting would lead to a blood loss exceeding 3000 ml [27, 28], significantly increasing intraoperative risks and the potential for adverse events, such as ischemia-reperfusion injury (IRI), coagulation disorder, and acute respiratory distress syndrome (ARDS). However, helping the patient get rid of all the nonviable tissue as soon as possible is essential to stabilize and improve the patient's condition. To this end, we propose a refined excision strategy that enables excision of more than 60% TBSA at one sitting while ensuring minimized intraoperative blood loss.

[Key Technical Points of the Proposed Strategy]

- **Preservation of interlayer tissue:** It is essential to preserve the interlayer tissue as much as possible. The interlayer here refers to the layer sandwiched between the uninjured underlying tissue and the definitely dead surface tissue. It is a transition layer that is compromised yet not dead. It has the potential to either survive or progress to complete necrosis during the patient's course.
- **Utilization of tourniquets:** Deploy tourniquets during extremity excision to help control blood loss.
- **Sequencing of excision procedures:** Prioritize excision of the extremities before proceeding with trunk excision to optimize patient safety and stability.

[The Strategy]

This strategic approach aims to balance the need for aggressive debridement with the imperative to maintain patient safety and stability throughout the surgical process.

I. **The timing and scope of operation**

The preferred timing for the extra-large but conservative excision approach is between the third and seventh days post-injury, when the patient's condition is relatively stabilized following the initial burn shock stage. The determination of the operation scope is based on a comprehensive assessment of the patient's overall clinical status and wound conditions. With the new excision modality, up to 60% TBSA can be excised in a single surgical session. The remaining deeper wounds can be excised in a subsequent procedure 2 ~ 3 days later. Importantly, excision of the extremities is performed prior to that of the trunk. This sequencing, combined with the application of tourniquets during extremity excision, helps minimize blood loss and optimize the safety of the subsequent surgical steps.

II. **Preoperative preparation**

1. **Stabilization of patient condition**

    1. A thorough medical history should be obtained to identify any underlying conditions that require treatment. An interdisciplinary approach may be implemented as needed.
    2. A comprehensive preoperative assessment, including various tests and examinations, is essential. The functions of vital organs such as the heart,

lungs, liver, and kidneys should be meticulously evaluated. Patients with large-area burns often experience hypoproteinemia due to the shock state, which can lead to pleural effusions and compromise surgical safety. This is particularly concerning in elderly patients and those with chronic lung conditions. Continuous monitoring of pleural effusions prior to surgery, along with measures to correct hypoproteinemia and enhance urine output, can significantly improve surgical safety.

3. Continuous efforts should be made to correct shock, anemia, and hypoproteinemia and to maintain water and electrolyte balance as well as acid-base balance.
4. Attention is also paid to improving the coagulation status. Patients with significantly reduced platelets should be supplemented with platelets; those with prolonged prothrombin time need to be corrected with transfusion of prothrombin complex, vitamin K1, etc.
5. For patients exhibiting multiple organ dysfunction since the shock stage, collaboration with anesthesiologists is essential to assess the impact of this dysfunction on the patient's tolerance for anesthesia and surgery, as well as to evaluate whether the operation may improve or exacerbate the dysfunction.
6. For patients with concomitant injuries, such as fractures or craniocerebral trauma, targeted examinations should be conducted to facilitate appropriate management, prioritizing treatment of the most critical conditions first. Once priorities are clarified, timely symptomatic treatment should be initiated to mitigate intraoperative risks.

2. **Management of blood loss and blood products**

Generally, blood loss from tangential excision or excision to the fat layer is greater than that from excision to the fascial layer. Traditionally, for adult patients, a minimum of 100 ml of blood is prepared for every 1% TBSA of extremities to be excised tangentially or the fat layer with the use of tourniquets, and at least 150 ml for every 1% TBSA of the trunk where tourniquets are not applicable. However, with the proposed strategy, preparation of at least 50 ml and 80 ml of blood for extremity and trunk excisions, respectively, is recommended. This is because the conservative approach preserves the inter-layer tissue as much as possible, contributing to an overall reduction in blood loss. For patients with decreased platelets, intraoperative platelet transfusions may be necessary and supplementation of coagulation factors or prothrombin complex may be indicated based on laboratory results.

3. **Infection prevention**

Upon admission, wound exudate and sputum samples should be collected for culture, and drug susceptibility testing should be ordered to identify the most effective antibiotics. Before the return of culture results, antibiotic selection should be guided by the bacteriological and epidemiological profiles pertinent to the burn center. Broad-spectrum antibiotics are typically employed in the early stages of the treatment course to cover both Gram-negative and Gram-positive bacteria. It is also emphasized that antibiotics should be administered simultaneously with the induction of anesthesia.

4. **Local wound and catheterization**

   1. Appropriate protection of the wounds to be excised is essential. Deep second-degree wounds should be properly dressed to prevent exacerbation of injury depth due to wound desiccation. Third-degree wounds should be left exposed, kept clean and dry, and treated with topical application of sulfadiazine silver or 1% iodine tincture to prevent wound infection and maceration.
   2. Proper dressing materials for temporary wound coverage should be prepared. For extra-large size but conservative excision, commercially available xenogeneic skin (e.g., porcine skin) is preferred.
   3. Deep venous and arterial catheters should be placed to ensure safe intraoperative fluid administration and reliable blood pressure monitoring. They will also facilitate intraoperative arterial blood gas analysis and timely adjustments.

5. **Additional considerations**

   1. The operating room temperature should be maintained at 37 °C.
   2. Both wound irrigation fluids and intravenous fluids should be adequately warmed prior to use.
   3. A clear airway should be ensured throughout the procedure, with heightened vigilance for elderly patients and those with chronic lung diseases. The necessity to strengthen intraoperative suctioning should be kept in mind.

III. **Intraoperative technical considerations**

1. **Excision depth control**

The strategy of extra-large size but conservative excision is designed to rid the patient of the definitely necrotic tissue as much as possible while minimizing intraoperative injury and blood loss by preserving the interlayer tissue. It should be noted that the preservation of the interlayer tissue in a large whole piece should be avoided and that preservation in a scattered pattern surrounded by the viable tissue is recommended. With this pattern, the excised wound surface typically exhibits scattered spots of bleeding and strips of fat tissue, indicating appropriate depth of excision. However, exposure of fat tissue in large, continuous areas may be necessary to ensure complete removal of devitalized tissue. When it is hard to determine the excision depth, visual inspection of traces of definitely viable tissue attached to the excised pieces can help guide the procedure.

2. **Free-hand dermatome technique**

With this strategy, excision is performed with a free-hand dermatome, which permits adjustment of the pressure, angle, and depth of the cutting blade based on the varying characteristics of the eschar. A tentative initial cut can be made when the optimal excision depth is difficult to determine. Then the screws are adjusted for proper thickness, and the eschar surface is tightened and smoothed out to ensure a neat operation. For concave surfaces, sub-eschar injection of a proper amount of normal saline can be helpful. A synchronous inspection of the underside of the cut eschar throughout the excision is needed to help the surgeon determine whether or not to adjust the operating pressure, knife angle, or the cutting depth. For areas with thinner skin, such as the dorsum of the hands or feet, fingers, and toes, particular caution is emphasized to avoid inadvertent exposure of deeper structures such as tendons or joints.

3. **Blood loss control**

During extremity excision, tourniquets are employed, and a complete hemostasis through ligation of large vessel breaks or electrocoagulation of smaller ones following excision is required. Diffuse bleeding can be treated with compression of warm gauze pads impregnated with saline or adrenaline in saline (5 μg/ml). For trunk excision, the pace of operation should be controlled to allow time for adequate hemostasis, avoiding excessive bleeding from overly rapid excision. To reduce bleeding, a proper amount of adrenaline in normal saline (1 μg/ml) can be injected under the eschar through adjacent healthy skin before excision. If no healthy skin is available, a portion of the eschar can be excised first and through the freshly excised surface, the solution can be injected to under the surrounding eschar. Should the patient's blood pressure be high during operation, the adrenaline solution can be replaced with normal saline.

4. **Biological dressing coverage**

Wounds excised with this strategy require coverage with proper dressings. Generally, the purchased xenogeneic skin (typically porcine skin) is preferred. Since xenogeneic skin grafts can easily dry and shrink, they should be placed along the body's vertical axis without any tension or sutures/staples, with adequate spacing between the graft pieces. Other biological dressings are also acceptable. For wounds with greater fat exposure or where allogeneic skin is available, allogeneic skin with vitality would be the optimal choice.

IV. **Postoperative care**

1. CBC and coagulation tests should be reordered 4 h postoperatively. Physicians should be alert to the possibility of severe anemia due to postoperative bleeding, particularly for patients with excision of the trunk, buttocks, or other areas that are difficult to compress and wrap.
2. For wounds covered with xenogeneic skin, which can readily dry and shrink, appropriate dressing techniques are essential to prevent rapid desiccation and the associated impact on wound healing. Additionally, close monitoring

of the patient's respiratory status and peripheral perfusion is necessary to detect and address any limitations in thoracic movement or compartment syndrome in the extremities due to the drying and shrinkage of the xenogeneic skin.

[Typical Case]

The patient was a 32-year-old gentleman with a history of hypertension who sustained scalds of 100% TBSA after accidentally falling into a cooling pool containing calcium oxide and silica (temperature approximately 72 °C; pH 9) at his workplace. Following the incident, he was immediately sent to a local hospital where he underwent tracheotomy and experienced acute renal dysfunction and oliguria that evening. He was subsequently referred to our center 23 h post-injury. Upon admission, the patient was lethargic but maintained clear consciousness and cooperated during physical examination. His total burn size was 100% TBSA, with third-degree burns exceeding 95% TBSA, primarily affecting both lower extremities. Deep second-degree burn wounds were noted mainly in the craniofacial region and the upper posterior trunk.

Admission diagnoses: ① Burn size: 100% TBSA (scald and chemical burns), deep second-degree (4%), third-degree (95%), fourth-degree (1%); ② acute kidney injury; ③ hypoproteinemia; ④ hypocalcemia; ⑤ coagulation abnormalities; ⑥ status post-tracheotomy; ⑦ hypertension.

Treatment course: Upon admission, vigorous anti-shock treatment was initiated. After careful evaluation of the patient's condition, an emergency excision was scheduled for the second day post-admission (the third day post-injury). The strategy of extra-large size but conservative excision was employed, targeting the four extremities and the anterior trunk. In preparation for the procedure, routine preoperative examinations were conducted, and fiberoptic bronchoscopy was performed to assess airway status. Thoracoscopy revealed pleural effusion on the left side with a depth of 0.5 cm. The plan for extensive excision was communicated with the anesthesia and blood transfusion teams to optimize preoperative preparation. Special attention was given to warming the operating room and ensuring the ventilator was functioning properly during the transfer from the ward to the operating room. Given the potential for significant exposure of fat tissue due to the depth of some wounds, a sufficient supply of allogeneic skin, in addition to commercially available porcine skin, was prepared. The operation proceeded smoothly, and the patient remained stable throughout. The excision was executed as planned, with a total excision size of 60% TBSA. Wounds that received tangential excision were covered with porcine skin, and those with deeper cuts, which left large patches of fat tissue exposed on the left upper extremity, were covered with allogeneic skin (Fig. 3.11). The patient's condition was stable following the first operation. Two days later (the fifth day post-injury), the same strategy was employed for the excision of the craniofacial area, posterior trunk, and buttocks, with a total size of approximately 20% TBSA. The excised wounds on the posterior trunk and buttocks were also covered with porcine

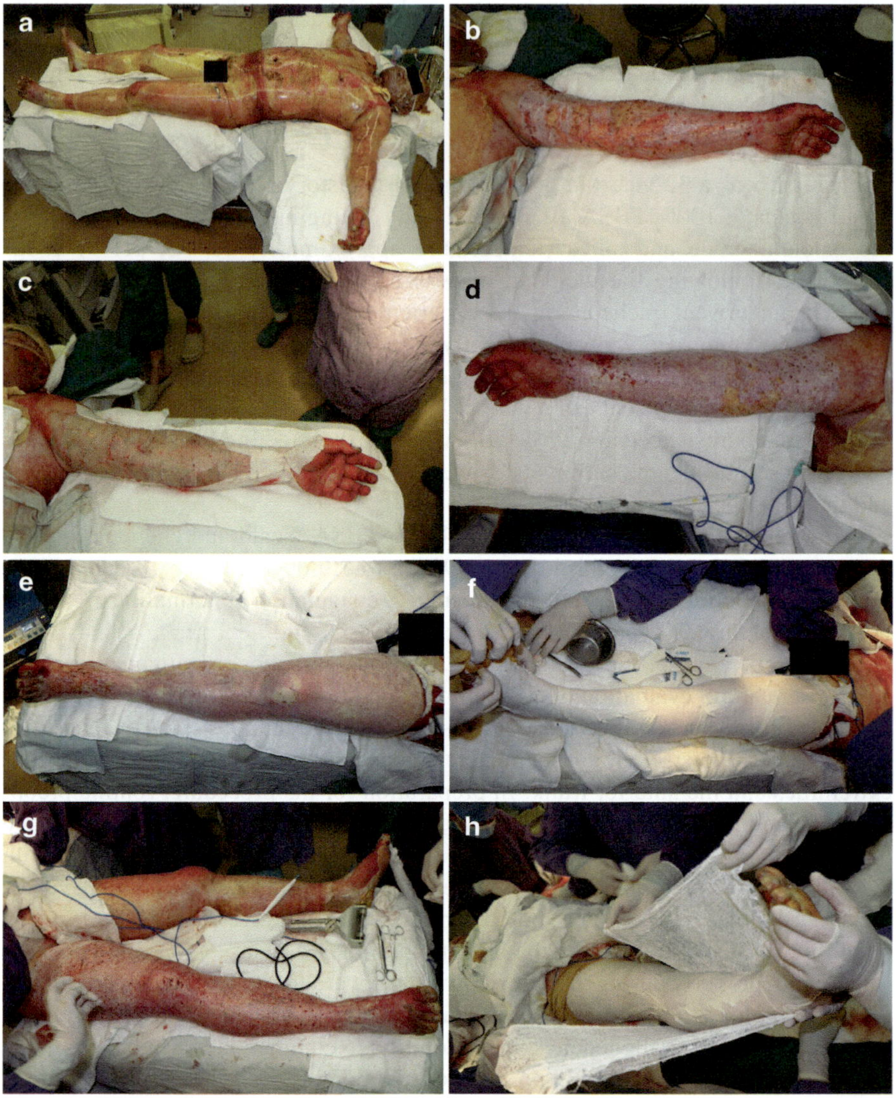

Fig. 3.11 The strategy of extra-large size but conservative excision was employed for the anterior trunk and the four extremities of a patient with 100%TBSA burn (60% TBSA was excised at one sitting). (**a**) Overall condition of the wounds. (**b**) Large patches of fat tissue were left exposed after excision (left upper extremity). (**c**) The exposed fat tissue on the left upper extremity was covered with allogeneic skin, and the rest of the wounds were dressed with porcine skin. (**d**) Excised wounds on the right upper extremity. (**e**) Excised wounds on the left lower extremity. (**f**) The debrided wounds on the left lower extremity were covered with porcine skin. (**g**) Excised wounds on the right lower extremity. (**h**) The debrided wounds on the right lower extremity were covered with porcine skin. (**i**) Anterior trunk wounds before excision. (**j**) Anterior trunk wounds after excision. (**k**) The debrided wounds on the anterior trunk were covered with porcine skin

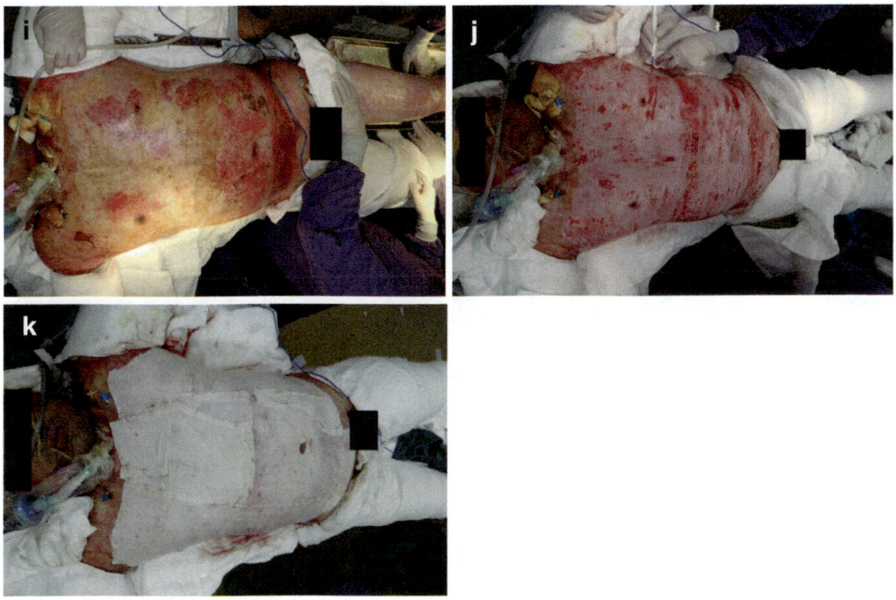

Fig. 3.11 (continued)

skin (Fig. 3.12). Collectively, these two procedures successfully removed necrotic tissue from wounds totaling about 80% TBSA. The patient's condition remained stable, with serum creatinine levels decreasing from 178% μmol/L at admission to approximately 76 μmol/L and procalcitonin levels dropping from 3.16 ng/ml to 0.475 ng/ml. Subsequently, wounds on the patient's head, posterior trunk, and buttocks partially healed with conservative treatment and served as donor sites for autologous skin grafting. Autografts, together with scalp grafts donated by relatives, were utilized to cover the residual wounds using the Meek technique and the intermingled transplantation of postage-stamp allo- and autografts. For illustrative purposes, the treatment course and outcomes for the left lower extremity are shown in Fig. 3.13. After 2 months, complete wound healing was achieved, and the skin regained functionality, supported by appropriate scar management and functional rehabilitation (Fig. 3.14).

[Discussion]

Previous studies have demonstrated that, in addition to the mass production of inflammatory mediators, a significant bacterial load can be present beneath necrotic tissue or eschar. This bacterial presence not only contributes to infection but also leads to a range of complications [29], including multi-system and organ dysfunction. Therefore, timely removal of necrotic tissue is critical for alleviating and stabilizing patient conditions [30, 31]. Traditionally, the extent of excision has been limited to 30% TBSA due to the associated risk of significant blood loss. While there are isolated reports of excisions extending to 60% TBSA at one sitting, such outcomes heavily depend on the skill and collaboration of the surgical team. In

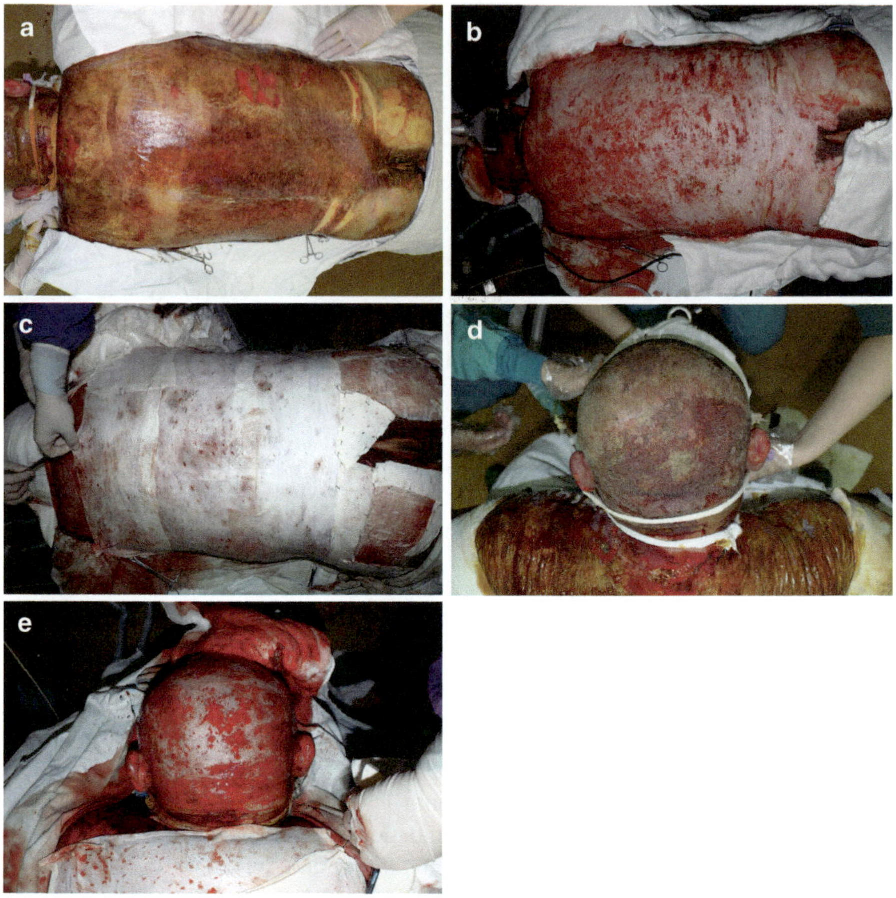

Fig. 3.12 The second operation was performed with the same excision strategy and rid the patient of necrotic tissue from another 20% TBSA of burn wounds on his head, posterior trunk, and buttocks. (**a**) Wounds on the posterior trunk and buttocks before excision. (**b**) Wounds on the posterior trunk and buttocks after excision. (**c**) The debrided wounds on the posterior trunk and buttocks were covered with porcine skin. (**d**) Scalp before excision. (**e**) Scalp after excision

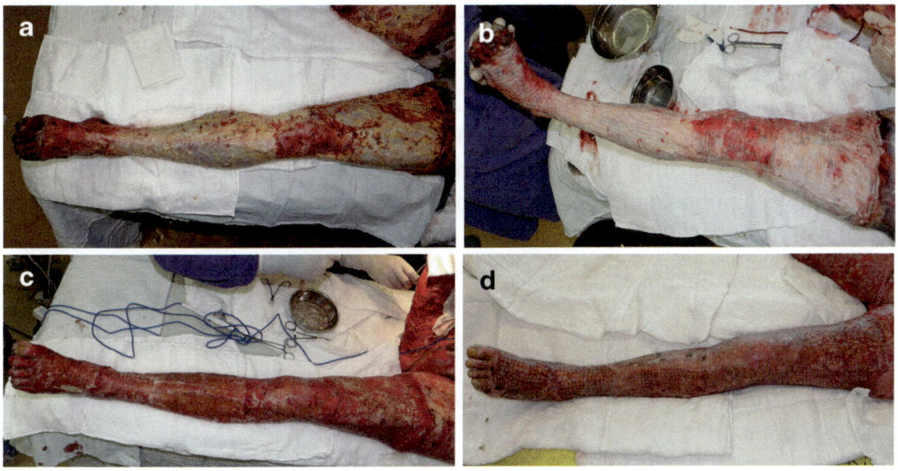

Fig. 3.13 Excision and outcomes of the patient's left lower extremity. (**a**) After the removal of the porcine skin on the left lower extremity, excision was repeated and reached the deep fascia layer to prepare a wound bed receptive to Meek grafts. (**b**) Meek grafting was performed for the left lower extremity. (**c**) Subsequent to the first Meek grafting, it could be seen that the microskin grafts grew and expanded, providing coverage for the majority of the wound surface. (**d**) Two months post-injury, the wounds on the left lower extremity healed, the visible evidence of Meek grafts expansion was apparent, and the overall skin texture was deemed satisfactory

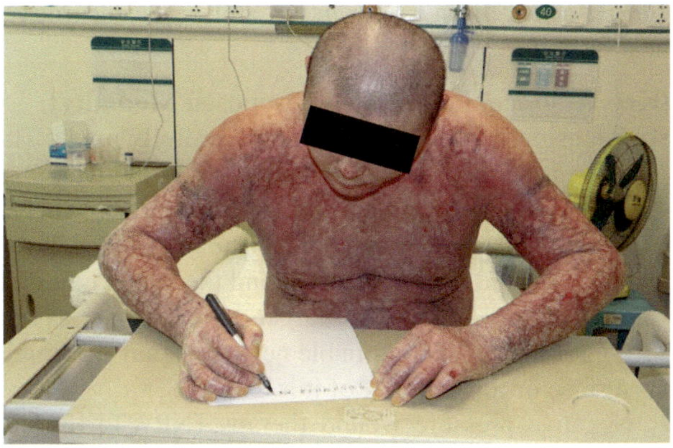

Fig. 3.14 The patient was instructed to do functional exercises upon wound healing

short, as excision size increases, both the blood loss and the associated risks rise accordingly. Therefore, minimizing blood loss has become a crucial factor in facilitating larger excisions.

The key of the extra-large size but conservative excision lies in "conservative," that is, to preserve the interlayer tissue while exposing healthy tissue. With this strategy, the amount of bleeding can be markedly reduced, which reduces the intraoperative risks and ensures the feasibility of extra-large size excision. On one hand, it allows for the removal of the majority of necrotic tissue, expediting the treatment process and stabilizing or even improving the patient's condition. On the other hand, it employs appropriate wound coverage to prepare the wound bed for subsequent autologous skin grafting.

This strategy has been clinically validated with positive treatment outcomes at our center. It requires straightforward techniques and can be effectively implemented by teams lacking advanced technical support. Therefore, this strategy presents a novel option for the management of patients with large burns, especially those with super extensive burns.

(Chuanan Shen, Jianhua Cai)

3.3.2 Phased Excision and Suture of Deep Burn Wounds

[Background]

The ideal conventional way to repair large deep burns is by autografting [32]. However, the harvesting of autografts may result in discoloration or scarring at the donor sites, and the grafted skin is susceptible to infection, hematoma formation, and potential failure to thrive. Even when successful engraftment occurs, the cosmetic result is often inferior to the normal skin. To improve the cosmetic results, we propose a new surgical modality, i.e., phased excision and suture of deep burn wounds. It is a modality that can directly minimize the wound surface area through cutting away the necrotic tissue and scars and then sewing up the surrounding healthy skin.

[Key Technical Points of the Proposed Modality]

- A tension-based excision plan is carefully made. The excision is performed in a phased manner due to the large size of the deep burn wound. The width of the wound surface that can be safely excised, as well as the direction of suturing, is determined by evaluating the tension of the local tissue. For smaller wounds, the entire wound may be excised and the surrounding healthy skin approximated at one sitting. However, for larger wounds, a series of sequential excisions, allowing for the growth of pliable new skin, may be anticipated until the entire wound surface or the majority of it is excised.
- Negative pressure wound therapy (NPWT) [33] is employed for the sutured wound, lasting for approximately 2 weeks. It reduces both wound tension and inflammatory exudate, thereby optimizing wound healing.

[The Modality]

I. **Indications and contraindications**

1. Indications:

   The proposed surgical approach can be employed for deep burn wounds on the trunk or extremities, particularly those surrounded by healthy skin that can be sutured following phased excision. Even in cases where complete excision is not feasible, as long as the wound tension permits, the modality still can be considered to minimize the wound surface area.

2. Contraindications

   1. Female patients who are pregnant, lactating, or menstruating
   2. Patients with uncontrolled hypertension
   3. Elderly patients with cardiopulmonary dysfunction
   4. Patients who are unable to strictly adhere to medical instructions
   5. Patients with wound infections

II. **Preoperative preparation**

Preoperative wound dressing changes play a crucial role in reducing local bacteria load, inflammatory response, and edema. A bacterial culture of the wound surface is necessary to determine the appropriate antibiotics. Patients with diabetes should have their blood sugar meticulously controlled. Prior to the operation, the wound size and tension of the local tissue are evaluated to determine potential suture directions and phases to be performed. ECG, CBC, urine analysis, and stool tests are requested. A preoperative interview is conducted to discuss with the patient the 2-week application of NPWT, as well as to inform the patient about the necessity of an extended suture length beyond the imaginary line of the long axis of the excised area, the possibility of dehiscence, and potential scar formation.

III. **Intraoperative procedures**

1. **Patient positioning**: Optimal exposure of the surgical site is achieved through proper patient positioning. For example, a prone position is recommended for wounds located on the calf, while a lateral position may be suitable for wounds on the lateral trunk or axilla. Additionally, patient positioning should aim to minimize tension in the wound area. For instance, a dorsal recumbent position is advised for wounds on the lower abdomen.
2. **Disinfection**: Wounds covered with dry scabs are typically disinfected using povidone-iodine. Wounds with excessive exudation or maceration should be washed with a sequential application of hydrogen peroxide solution, povidone-iodophor solution, and gentamicin-containing saline after anesthesia and before disinfection. This protocol helps prevent wound bacteria from contaminating the surgical field.
3. **Wound excision**: The proposed modality aims to achieve improved cosmetic outcomes; therefore, minimal tension along the suture should be obtained while performing approximation. Measures to minimize such tension include parallelization of the cut to the skin lines when feasible and proper positioning of target joints to minimize tension in the affected area. Generally, for small wounds that can be excised at one sitting, the incision is carried 1–2 millimeters away from the edge of the necrotic tissue, extending vertically to the fat layer, and for deeper wounds with fat tissue necrosis, to the level of the deep fascia. Whereas for large wounds requiring phased

excision, the incision is carried within the wound area. For large extremity wounds, the excision should be performed with the assistance of tourniquets after exsanguination. For large trunk wounds, the injection of an appropriate amount of adrenaline-containing saline (1 μg/m) beneath the wound prior to excision is recommended to reduce bleeding. Electrocoagulation is performed to stop bleeding from small blood vessels, while ligation is used for larger ones. Care should be taken to protect the skin edge from repeated pulling or pinching by surgical instruments. The length of approximation is often greater than half of the perimeter of the wound. For the central surgical area under high tension, it is recommended to conduct an intradermal suture followed by a simple interrupted suture superficially. If skin tension allows, scars formed on the wound edges can also be excised to improve cosmetic appearance. For wounds with exceptionally high tension, selective dissociation can be performed bilaterally from the incision line at the deep fascial level to reduce tension. For large-size and deep excisions, a Penrose drain or negative pressure drainage tube can be placed and discontinued 3 to 4 days after surgery.

4. **Suture following tension reduction and fixation**: The following techniques can be employed to minimize skin tension during suturing. First, a cut is made at the deep fascia level with bilateral dissociation to reduce local tension. Second, layered suturing, in which subcuticular absorbable stitches and mattress suture to reduce and distribute tension evenly, is adopted. Finally, NPWT is added to further reduce skin tension. Films are used to pull the skin from both sides in opposite directions, redistributing tension away from the incision edge. Then the negative pressure devices are sealed, and suction is initiated to ensure that the incision heals under a relaxed, tension-free condition.

IV. **Postoperative care**

Optimal antibiotic therapy is tailored to individual patients following bacterial culture results. Proper patient positioning is crucial to minimize wound tension and enhance healing. Vigilant monitoring of circulatory status in bandaged extremities, including arms, legs, hands, and feet, is imperative. Close supervision of negative pressure wound therapy is essential, maintaining negative pressure within the range of 0.02–0.04 MPa. Between the second and fourth days post-surgery, the outer dressings are removed to inspect the negative pressure suction devices. Any torn films or those showing air leaks should be promptly replaced. In cases where the negative pressure tubes are obstructed by blood clots, flushing with normal saline is recommended. Caution must be exercised to prevent excessive solution from entering the negative pressure apparatus and dampening the wound environment. Typically, negative pressure wound therapy is discontinued 10–12 days post-surgery, after which sutures are retained, and proper positions or tapes are employed for continuous tension reduction.

Adequate joint fixation is essential for closures near or at joints. Suture removal is generally scheduled for the 14th day post-surgery; however, certain stitches may be left in place longer based on wound tension and healing progress to prevent potential closure dehiscence.

[Typical Case]

The patient was a 26-year-old woman who sustained multiple flame burns on the face, abdomen, and all four extremities at her home in Melbourne, at 5:00 am on October 30, 2019. She was found unconscious by firefighters and subsequently transported to a local medical center. During transportation, she received emergency tracheal intubation and ventilatory support. At the center, she underwent excision and skin grafting procedures four times, but the graft survival rate was low. On December 11, 2019 (42 days post-injury), the patient was referred to our center with complaints of multiple flame burns and refractory wounds.

Specialized physical exams: The total burn size of the wounds on the face, anterior trunk, and four extremities was approximately 13% TBSA. Some of the wounds had already healed, with formation of darker-colored and tougher-textured scars. The nonhealing wounds accounted for approximately 4% TBSA and were located on the abdomen and four extremities. These wounds exhibited desiccated, shrunken, and necrotic fat tissue without any signs of bleeding. The back of the right hand and right forearm exhibited necrotic eschars, exposed tendons, stiff joints, and limited mobility. Mild scar formation and pigmentation were observed at the donor sites on the back and right thigh.

Admission diagnoses: ① Multiple unhealed burn wounds: size, 4%TBSA; depth, third- to fourth-degree; ② infected wounds; ③ multiple scars; ④ hypoglobulinemia; ⑤ anemia.

Treatment course: After admission, the patient received debridement, dressing changes, bath therapy, laser therapy, administration of human immunoglobulin, anti-infection therapy, and nutritional support. The patient opposed skin grafting because she felt anxious about this treatment due to the poor survival rate of the grafts in her previous surgeries. In view of this, the phased excision and suture approach was chosen for the unhealed wounds. The first operation was performed on December 18, 2019, during which residual wounds and scars on both lower extremities, left upper extremity, and abdomen were partially excised and sutured under general anesthesia. The second operation was performed on January 21, 2020, involving partial excision and suturing of scars in the bilateral subcostal and facial areas, as well as debridement and autologous grafting of residual wounds on the right upper extremity and abdomen under general anesthesia. The third operation was performed on February 20, 2020, under general anesthesia, with further partial excision and suturing of scars on both lower extremities, left upper extremity, and abdomen. All surgically treated wounds received negative pressure wound therapy. For wounds that had been completely excised, NPWT was maintained for 13 days, whereas for those requiring phased excision, NPWT should be replaced in

Table 3.2 The size of wounds and scars after three operations and comparison with the admission data

Point in time	Size of wounds and scars (cm^2)				
	Left upper extremity	Abdomen	Left lower extremity	Total size[a]	Proportion[b]
Upon admission	203.50	209	376	1598.50	100%
After the first operation	122.75	152	70	1126.75	70.5%
After the second operation	122.75	127	170	1083.75	67.8%
After the third operation	77.75	101.5	101	812.75	50.8%

[a]The total size was added up from the sizes of wounds and scars on the face, four extremities, and anterior trunk. The table only presents the data from the left upper extremity, abdomen, and left lower extremity

[b]Proportion = the total size of the residual wounds and scars/the total size of the wounds and scars upon admission ×100%

1 week. Following the three operations, the patient's wounds were successfully closed, and the total size of the wounds and scars was halved (Table 3.2). Subsequently, the patient underwent rehabilitation treatments such as scar management and functional exercises and was eventually discharged on March 10, 2020 (see image sets in Fig. 3.15).

[Discussion]

In the above case, the local medical center initially suspected the presence of underlying autoimmune diseases contributing to the failure of skin grafting and the persistence of refractory wounds. Upon consultation at our facility, the patient expressed opposition to additional skin grafting. Consequently, we opted for the phased

Fig. 3.15 The modality of phased excision and suture for deep wounds was employed for a 26-year-old woman with multiple flame burns and previously refractory wounds. The first set of images showing the treatment course and outcome of the wounds and scars on the lower abdomen. (**a**) Previously refractory wounds and scars on the abdomen upon admission. (**b**) Excision during the first operation. (**c**) The excised areas were approximated and sutured during the first operation. (**d**) NPWT was employed following the first operation. (**e**) 23 days after the first operation. (**f**) Debridement during the second operation. (**g**) The debrided abdominal wound was grafted during the second operation. (**h**) NPWT was utilized following the second operation. (**i**) 13 days after the second operation. (**j**) Excision during the third operation. (**k**) The two sides on the opening were approximated and sutured during the third operation. (**l**) NPWT was utilized following the third operation. (**m**) 18 days after the third operation, the previously refractory wounds on the abdomen eventually healed and the wound size halved (101.5 cm^2 now vs. 209 cm^2 upon admission), improving both the patient condition and the cosmetic outcome

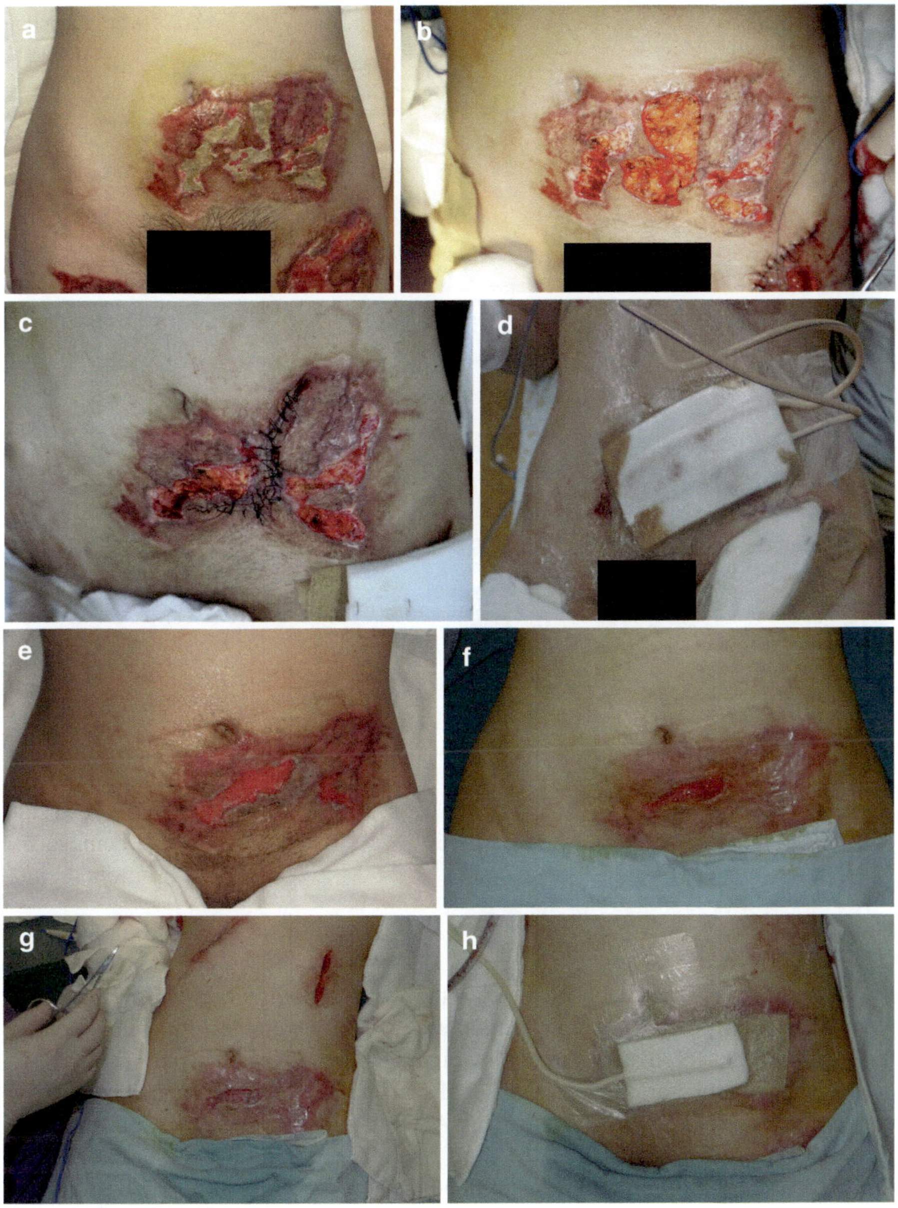

Fig. 3.15 (continued)

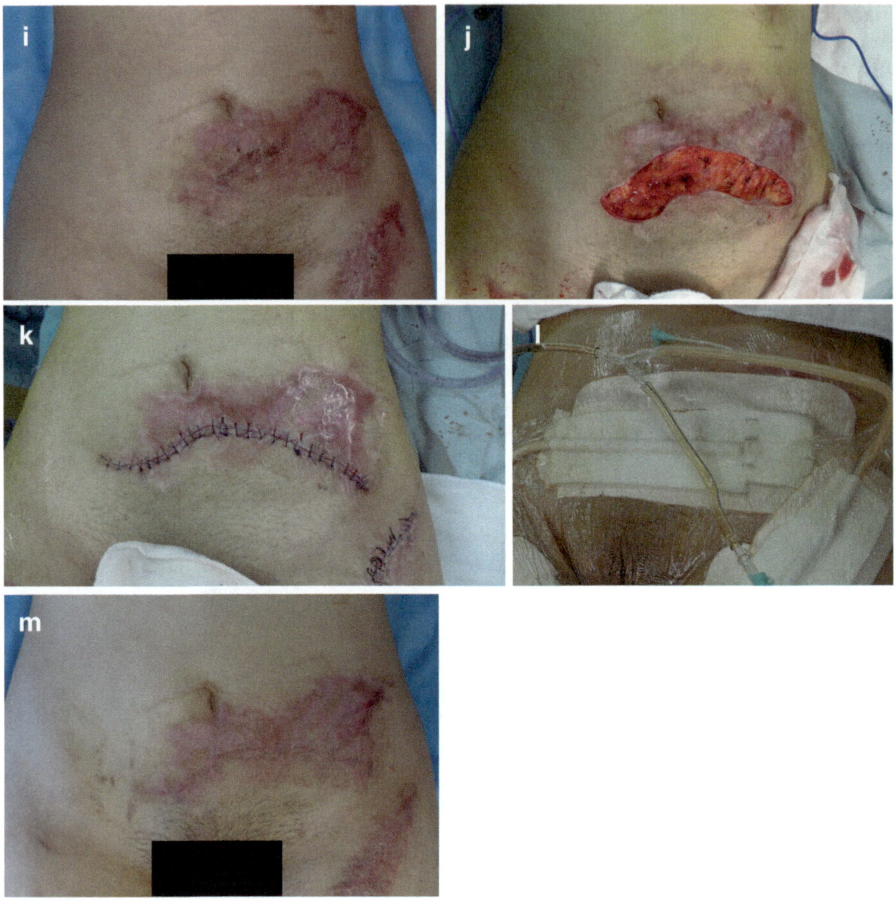

Fig. 3.15 (continued)

excision and suture approach to close all the wounds comprehensively. During the wound excision process, certain scars were also removed, resulting in a notable reduction in the overall scar size upon wound healing (Figs. 3.16 and 3.17).

After the first operation, the total size of scars and wounds was reduced to 70.5% of the initial measurement at admission. After the second operation, this size was further reduced to 67.8%. After the third operation, it diminished significantly to just 50.8% of the initial measurement at admission, as outlined in Table 3.2. Upon discharge, the patient reported no symptoms of pain or itching in the healed region. The approach demonstrates considerable benefits in terms of shortening treatment duration, enhancing cosmetic outcomes, and reducing long-term costs associated with scar management.

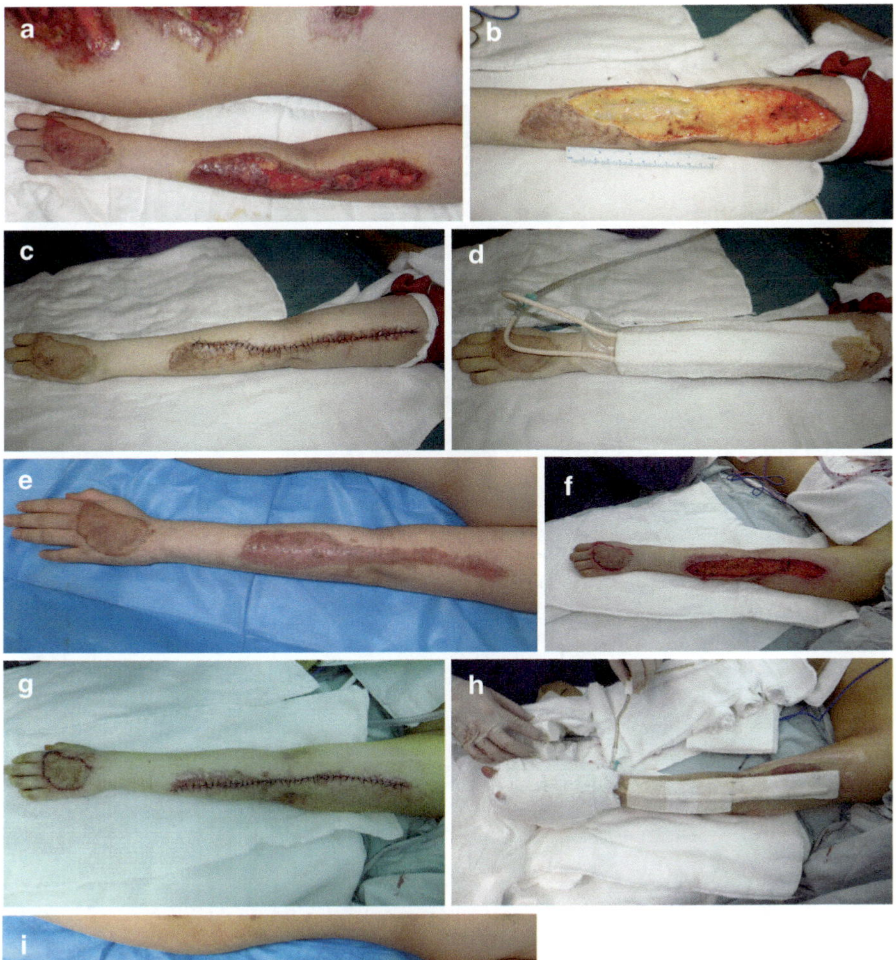

Fig. 3.16 The second set of images of the same patient illustrating the treatment course and outcome of the wounds and scars on the left upper extremity. (**a**) Previously refractory wounds and scars on the left upper extremity upon admission. (**b**) Excision during the first operation. (**c**) The two sides of the excised area were approximated and sutured during the first operation. (**d**). NPWT was utilized following the first operation. (**e**) 23 days after the first operation. (**f**) Scar excision during the second operation. (**g**) Approximation and suture were repeated during the second operation. (**h**) NPWT was utilized following the second operation. (**i**) 18 days after the second operation, the previously refractory wounds on the left upper extremity healed and the wound size was reduced to 122.75 cm^2 from 203.50 cm^2 upon admission

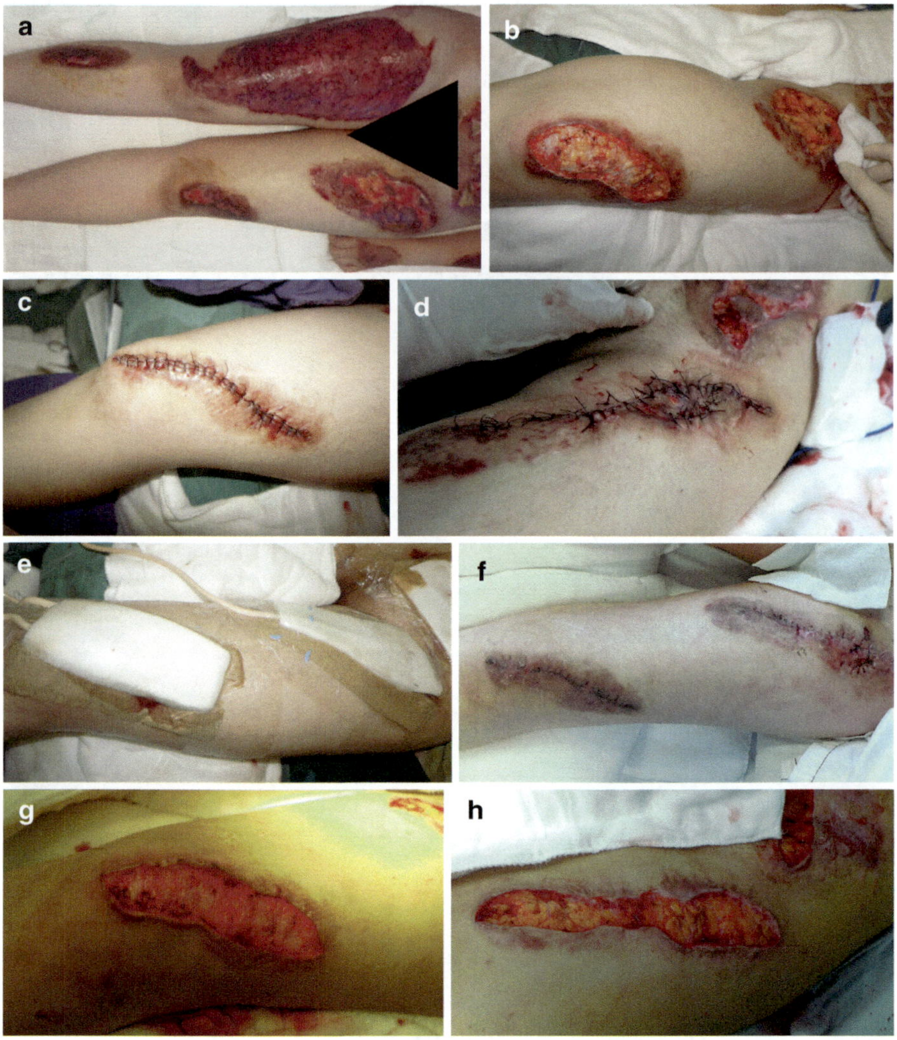

Fig. 3.17 The third set of images of the same patient illustrating the treatment course and outcome of the wounds and scars on the left lower extremity. (**a**) Previously refractory wounds and scars on the left lower extremity upon admission. (**b**) Excision of the wounds and scars on the left lower extremity during the first operation. (**c**) Approximation and suture of the excised wound overlying the left knee. (**d**) Approximation and suture of the excised wound on the left thigh. (**e**) NPWT was utilized following the first operation. (**f**) 23 days after the first operation. (**g**) Scar excision in the left knee area during the second operation. (**h**) Scar excision in the left thigh area during the second operation. (**i**) Suture in the left knee area during the second operation. (**j**) Suture in the left thigh area during the second operation. (**k**) NPWT was utilized following the second operation. (**l**) 18 days after the second operation

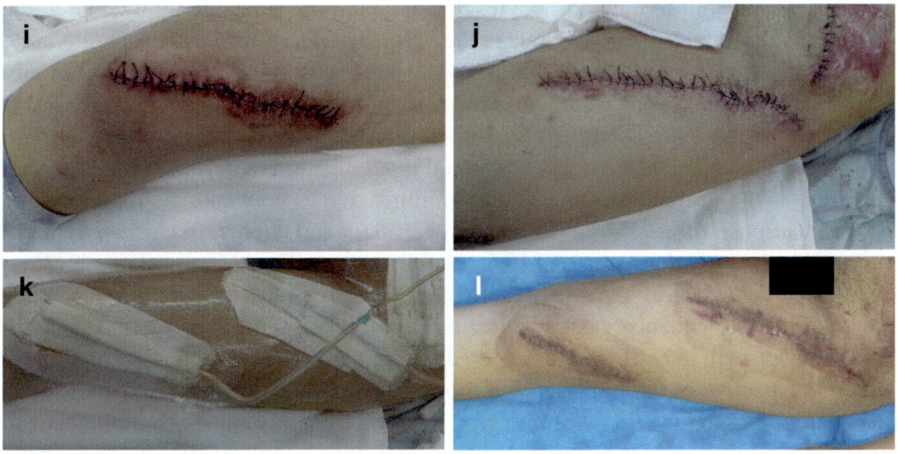

Fig. 3.17 (continued)

The phased excision and suture approach integrates multiple therapeutic interventions for wound repair and reconstruction in a comprehensive manner. Central to this approach is the incorporation of tension-reducing techniques within the surgical site, with the utilization of NPWT playing a pivotal role [34]. Its mechanism encompasses several key functions: ① Facilitating tension transfer and dispersion, thereby alleviating tension at the closure site and establishing a tension-free environment conducive to healing; ② efficient drainage of exudate and blood through continuous negative pressure suction, thereby minimizing the risk of infection; ③ the localized negative pressure aids in aligning the closure edges appropriately, promoting optimal wound healing outcomes.

(Chuanan Shen, Huping Deng)

3.3.3 Wound Type-Based Grafting

[Background]

Typically, excised wounds without substantial thickness loss can be categorized into two types: those retaining adipose tissue and those with residual dermal tissue. These distinct wound types create diverse environments for skin grafts, directly influencing the graft take rate [35]. Consequently, tailored skin grafting strategies for different wound types are essential to enhance graft viability, minimize graft consumption, and expedite wound healing.

Wounds with mixed burn depths may expose either adipose tissue or dermal tissue following excision. On surfaces that retain dermal tissue, autologous skin grafts are more likely to thrive and grow, whereas their success rate is diminished on surfaces with exposed adipose tissue. Notably, white adipose tissue primarily comprises clusters of white adipocytes, each containing a sizable lipid droplet that displaces the cytoplasm and nucleus to the periphery. The clusters are separated into lobules by thin layers of loose connective tissue, with minimal intercellular substance and limited vasculature. Moreover, adipose tissue vascularity decreases in obese individuals [36]. Direct application of microautologous skin grafts to adipose surfaces yields inferior outcomes compared to application to dermal or deep fascial surfaces, as the grafts are prone to non-viability due to poor blood supply and the exposed adipose tissue would desiccate, necrotize, and even suffer invasive infection in the absence of coverage of biological dressings. Therefore, utilizing biological dressings, such as allogeneic or xenogeneic skin, to prepare fat-retaining wounds can significantly enhance graft survival by promoting vascularization and granulation tissue growth [37]. It should be noted that though complete excision of adipose tissue irrespective of the burn depth, followed by application of microskin grafts to the deep fascia, may yield favorable graft survival rate, this approach often leads to pronounced hypertrophic scarring and contractures, compromising both aesthetic appearance and functionality [38].

In recent years, our team performed tailored skin grafting procedures based on the two types of the excised wounds, applying allogeneic or xenogeneic skin to the adipose surfaces for wound preparation and Meek autografting to the dermal surfaces [35]. This wound type-based grafting strategy has consistently delivered exceptional performance and yielded satisfactory outcomes.

[Protocol]

I. Indications

The strategy is suitable for patients with large deep burns who lack sufficient sources of autologous skin and have excised wounds that retain both healthy adipose tissue and dermal tissue.

II. Preoperative preparation

The size of deep second-degree wounds and third-degree wounds should be carefully evaluated. Roughly, the size of deep second-degree corresponds to the size of dermal tissue that will remain after excision, while the size of third-degree wounds corresponds to the adipose tissue that can be retained. Accordingly, adequate allo- or xenogeneic skin and Meek packs are prepared.

III. Surgical method

1. Excision is carried to the level of healthy tissue.
2. The excised wound is thoroughly rinsed after complete hemostasis.
3. After excision, the size of the adipose surface and the dermal surface is carefully measured with the Rule of Nine, wherein the dorsum of the patient's hand approximates 1% of the total body surface.
4. A proper amount of adrenaline-containing normal saline is injected subcutaneously at the donor site, autologous skin harvested, and Meek autografts fabricated.
5. The prepared allo- or xenogeneic skin is employed to cover the reserved adipose tissue, whereas the Meek autografts are transplanted to cover the reserved dermal tissue.

6. After grafting, the wounds are dressed with mesh gauze impregnated with sulfadiazine silver powder, followed by multiple layers of sterile gauze and gauze pads.
7. The outer layers of gauzes are removed within 1 week; the status of the Meek grafts and evidence of hematoma and exudates under the grafts are inspected, and the allo- or xenogeneic grafts are renewed if necessary.
8. Generally, in 2–3 weeks, the autologous skin islands in the Meek grafts would grow and fuse, while the adipose surface under the allo- or xenogeneic grafts would granulate [39]. Debridement is repeated, after which autografting is performed.

[Typical Case]

The patient, a 51-year-old woman, suffered multiple burns resulting from an LPG explosion and was admitted to our center approximately 5 h post-injury.

Admission diagnoses: ① Burn size, 92%TBSA; 2% TBSA, comprising 2% TBSA superficial second-degree burns, 20% TBSA deep second-degree burns, and 70% TBSA deep third-degree burns; ② severe inhalation injury; ③ burn shock.

Treatment course: The first operation was performed 5 days following the injury. During the operation, excision for the wounds on the right upper and the left lower extremities was performed, split-thickness skin grafts from the left upper and right lower extremities were harvested, adipose areas were covered with porcine skin, and dermis-retaining areas received Meek autografting. By the 21st day post-injury, robust reepithelialization was noted in the wounds treated with Meek autografting, and wounds covered with porcine skin showed healthy granulation. On the 25th day post-injury, postage-stamp autografts were transplanted onto the residual wounds with fresh granulation beds (Fig. 3.18).

[Discussion]

The essence of this technique lies in differentiated treatment based on different depths of wounds. Excised wounds retaining dermal tissue can benefit from direct application of Meek autografts, achieving earlier healing than those awaiting preparation. Conversely, those with residual fat are not suitable for Meek autografts, and to optimize autograft usage, these wounds can be temporarily covered with allo- or xenogeneic skin to promote wound vascularization and granulation for approximately 2 weeks before autografting. Attention should be paid to:

1. Perforation of the allogeneic or xenogeneic skin for improved exudate drainage
2. Scheduled dressing removal around 1 week postoperative for inspection of coverage integrity, exudates presence, with bacterial culture for abnormal exudation, and early dressing changes for noticeable exudation
3. Debridement of fat tissue to the level of healthy fat in fat-retaining areas

For patients with extensive burns, preserving unaffected skin is paramount and warrants cautious utilization. Surgeons must balance functional and cosmetic outcomes. Two approaches are cautioned against:

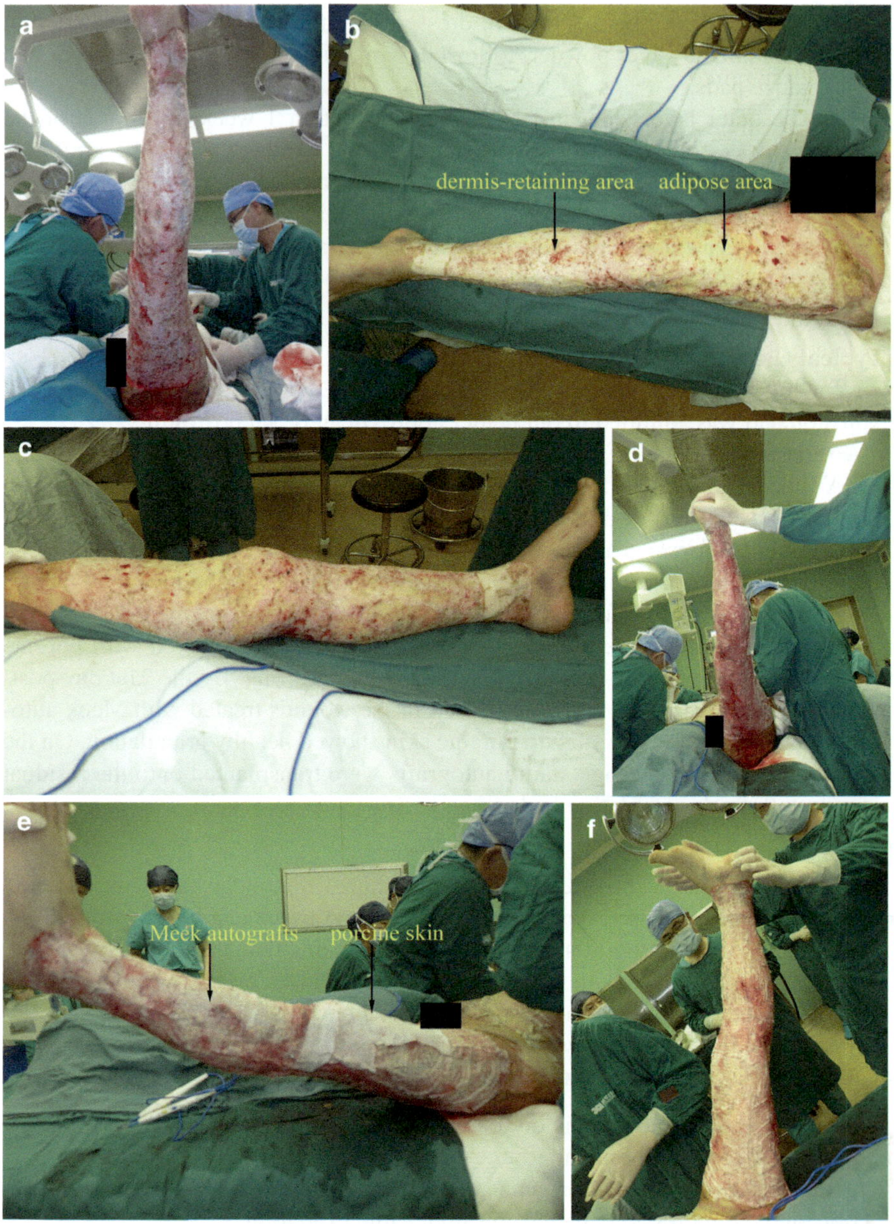

Fig. 3.18 A 92%TBSA burn patient treated with the wound type-based grafting strategy. (**a–c**) Posterior, anterior, and lateral views of the left lower extremity post-excision. (**d–f**) Excised left lower extremity covered with porcine skin in the adipose area and Meek autografts in the dermis-retaining area. (**g–i**) Following the previous treatment, the left lower extremity was observed with reepithelialization in the Meek grafting area and granulation in the porcine skin covered area. (**j–l**) The residual and granulated wounds on the extremity received Meek autografting

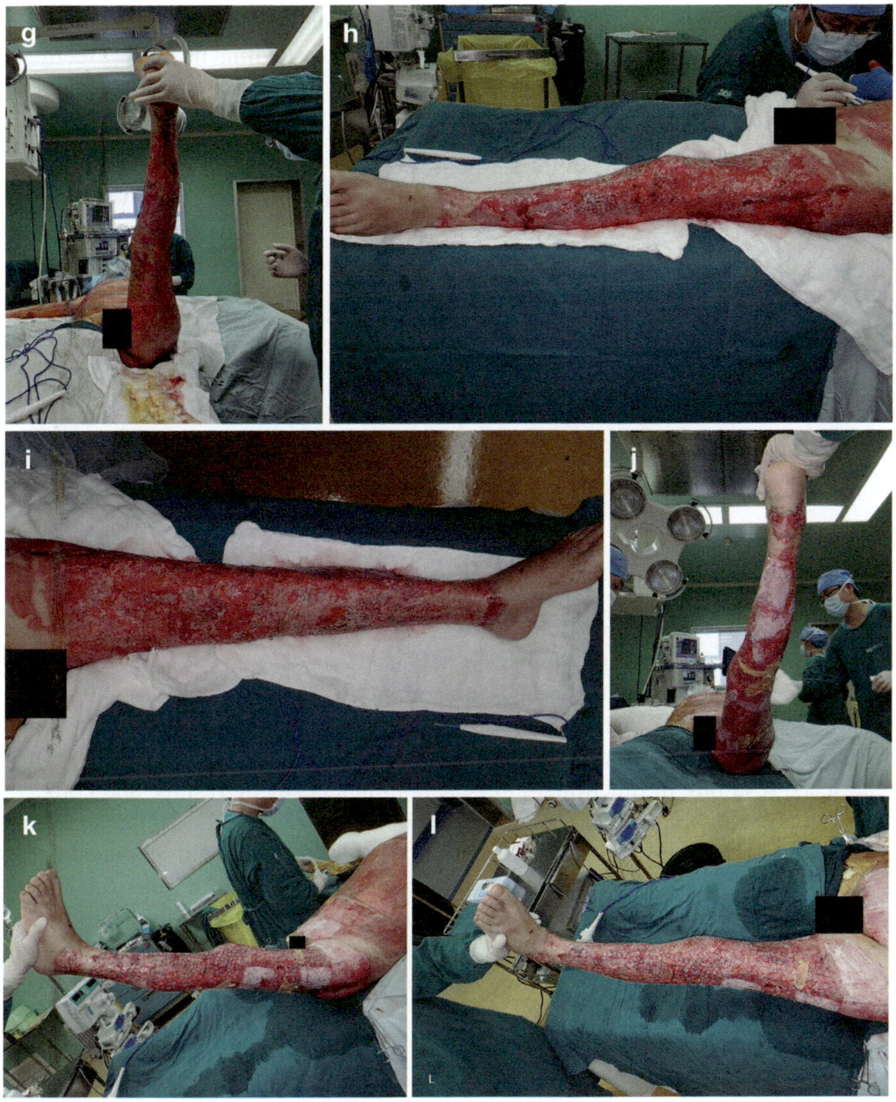

Fig. 3.18 (continued)

1. Universal Meek grafting for all wounds risks inadequate vascular supply to fat tissue, leading to necrosis and desiccation, potentially inviting invasive infections.
2. Overzealous debridement risks sacrificing functional and cosmetic benefits of retained fat tissue.

Careful evaluation and varied treatment for burns of different depths are essential. Preparing wounds for vascularization and granulation can conserve precious autologous skin. In essence, this strategy customizes treatments for diverse wound types, optimizes autografting, and offers a precise solution for managing extensive burn wounds.

(Chuanan Shen, Dongjie Li)

3.3.4 Wound Location-Specific Grafting

[Background]
In addition to life-saving efforts, the management of large or extensive burns necessitates comprehensive consideration of preventing hypertrophic scar formation and contracture. This is crucial for achieving optimal functional and aesthetic outcomes, particularly in areas involving joints.

Expanded skin grafting techniques are commonly employed in the management of large or extensive burns, as they enhance graft utilization and wound coverage efficiency [40]. However, these techniques can lead to the development of hypertrophic scars, resulting in functional limits, suboptimal cosmetic results, and compromised quality of life for the patient. Clinical observations indicate that scar and contracture formation may begin even before wound closure with expanded skin grafting, and their severity increases upon wound healing, making subsequent procedures such as releases and reconstructions more challenging, especially when deeper structures like blood vessels, nerves, tendons, and joints undergo irreversible changes [41]. Therefore, scar prevention should also be a primary consideration during the skin grafting process [42].

In this regard, the author proposes a strategy that entails differentiated grafting treatments for deep burn wounds at various sites during the early stage, taking into account the specific locations of the wounds [43]. When sufficient autologous skin is available, large sheets of thick split-thickness autograft are preferred for wounds overlying joints, while smaller autograft pieces can be employed in expanded grafting for wounds in other areas [44]. This approach ensures grafting efficiency and facilitates comprehensive functional restoration of joint areas in a single step, ultimately contributing to an improved overall recovery for patients with large or extensive burns [45].

[Protocol]

I. **Indications**

The strategy is applicable to large or extensive deep burns where residual autologous skin is available and can be harvested in sheets for the coverage of the joint areas.

II. **Preoperative preparation**

The sizes of the wounds that will undergo debridement are measured, with specific attention to assessing the circumference and length of the involved joint areas to determine the required autograft sheet size. The depths of these wounds are also assessed to inform the determination of skin harvest depths, since following debridement, deep second-degree burns typically retain partial dermal tissue, while third-degree burns expose fat tissue or the deep fascia. Subsequently, skin harvesting tools and an appropriate quantity of Meek crepes are readied.

III. **Intraoperative procedures**

1. Excision and debridement: Tailored excision is performed to various levels based on the depth of the wounds, with a focus on preserving viable fat tissue as much as possible in the joint areas to optimize functional restoration.
2. Complete hemostasis and irrigation.
3. Reassessment of the circumference and length of the involved joint area, followed by delineation of the area for autograft sheet harvesting at the donor site.
4. Estimation of non-joint area sizes with the Rule of Nine, wherein the dorsum of the patient's hand approximates 1% of the total body surface, to gauge the size of the autografts for expanded grafting in these areas.
5. Subcutaneous injection of epinephrine-containing saline into the autologous skin donor sites to facilitate the harvest of thick split-thickness autograft sheets for joint area coverage and thin split-thickness autografts for expanded grafting.
6. Perforation of the autograft sheets occurs following repeated rinsing with normal saline, while thin split-thickness autografts are prepared in large pieces, squares, postage-stamp skin grafts, or Meek grafts.
7. Application of the autograft sheet to the wound overlying the joint area, followed by fixation with staples.
8. Application of corresponding grafts to the remaining wounds.
9. Coverage of all grafted sites with a layer of mesh gauze soaked in sulfadiazine silver powder, over which multiple layers of sterile gauze and gauze pads are applied and secured.
10. One week later, the dressings are opened for inspection and the outer sterile gauze renewed. Sutures and staples typically can be removed by the tenth postoperative day.

[Typical Case]

The patient, a 32-year-old man, was admitted to our center 5 hours after sustaining multiple burns from an LPG explosion.

Admission diagnoses: ① Burns to multiple body parts, with a total burn size of 72% TBSA; deep second-degree, 16% TBSA; third-degree, 56% TBSA; ② severe inhalation injury; ③ post-tracheotomy.

Treatment course: During the first operation, the patient underwent excision on both lower extremities, autograft harvesting from donor sites on the head and left lower extremity, autograft sheet grafting for the left knee area, and Meek grafting for the remaining areas. The condition of the patient's lower extremities before operation is shown in Fig. 3.19.

After excision (Fig. 3.20), the left knee area was measured with an upper circumference of 38 cm, a lower circumference of 34 cm, and a distance of 10 cm between the two edges. A thick split-thickness autograft sheet measuring 35 cm by 10 cm was harvested from the available donor site on the lateral aspect of the right thigh using an electric dermatome (Fig. 3.21). After meticulous cleaning and perforation, the autograft sheet was carefully applied to the left knee area (Fig. 3.22). The remaining excised wounds on the left extremity were covered with Meek autografts (expansion ratio, 1:6). Three weeks after the operation, reepithelialization of the wounds with the Meek autografts and healing of the knee area with the autograft sheet were observed (Figs. 3.23 and 3.24). Follow-up examinations revealed satisfactory functionality and appearance of the knee (Fig. 3.25).

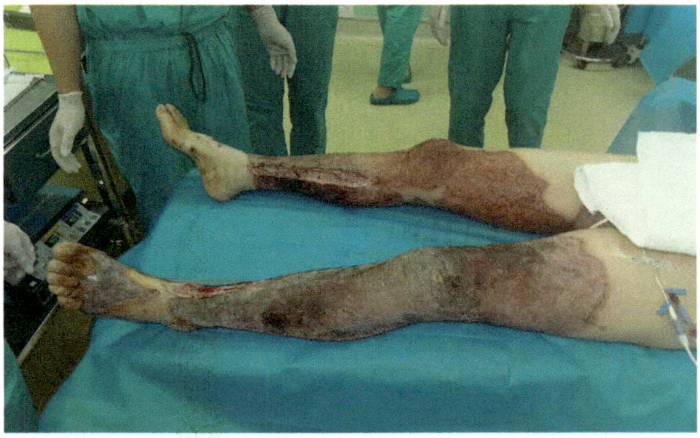

Fig. 3.19 The patient's lower extremities with eschar coverage before operation

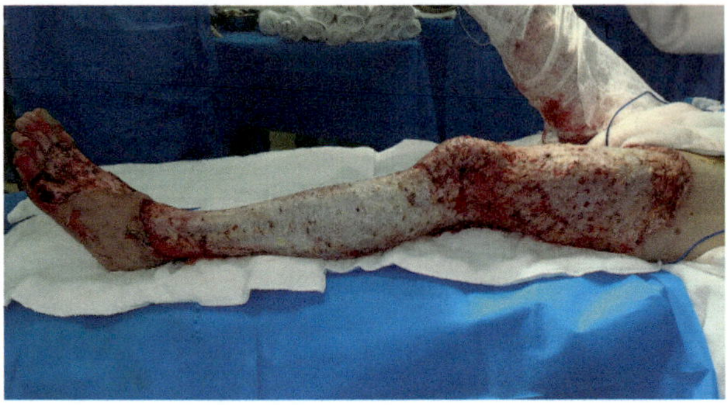

Fig. 3.20 The left lower extremity after excision

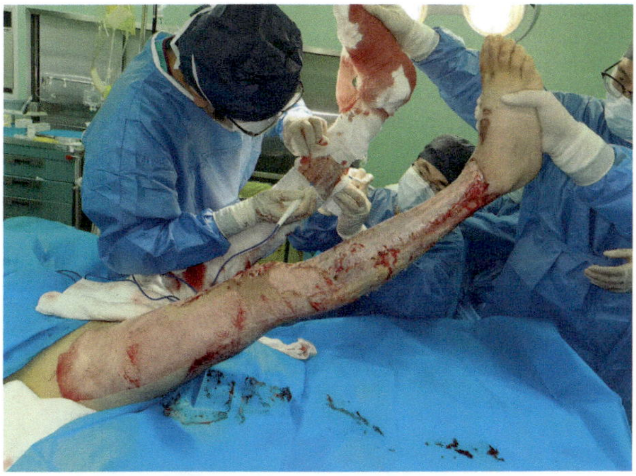

Fig. 3.21 Autograft sheets are harvested from the anterior and lateral aspects of the right thigh

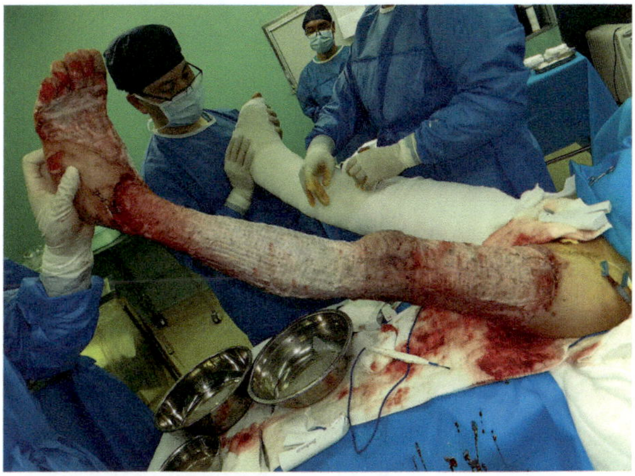

Fig. 3.22 The left knee area was covered with an autograft sheet harvested from the right thigh, and the remaining wounds of the left leg were covered with Meek autografts

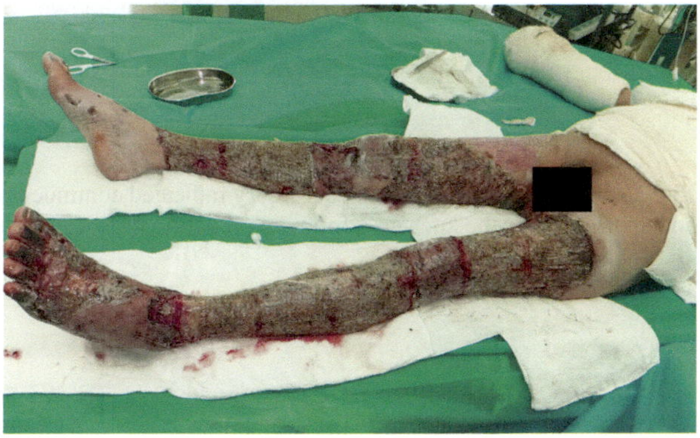

Fig. 3.23 Appearance of the grafted sites 3 weeks post-grafting

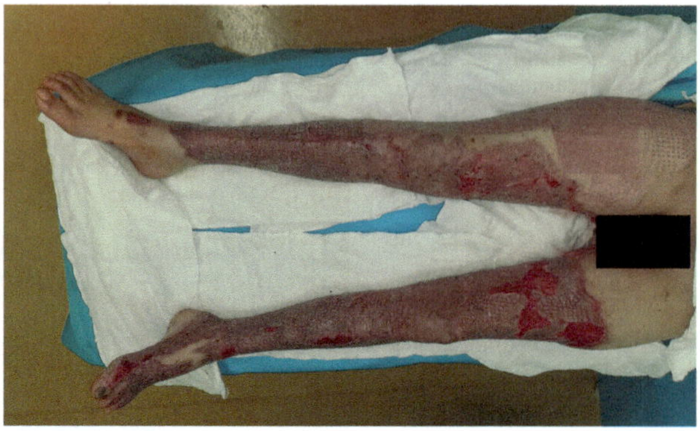

Fig. 3.24 The autograft sheet exhibited favorable growth, and the functional and aesthetic outcomes of the knee area were deemed satisfactory at the 4-week post-grafting assessment

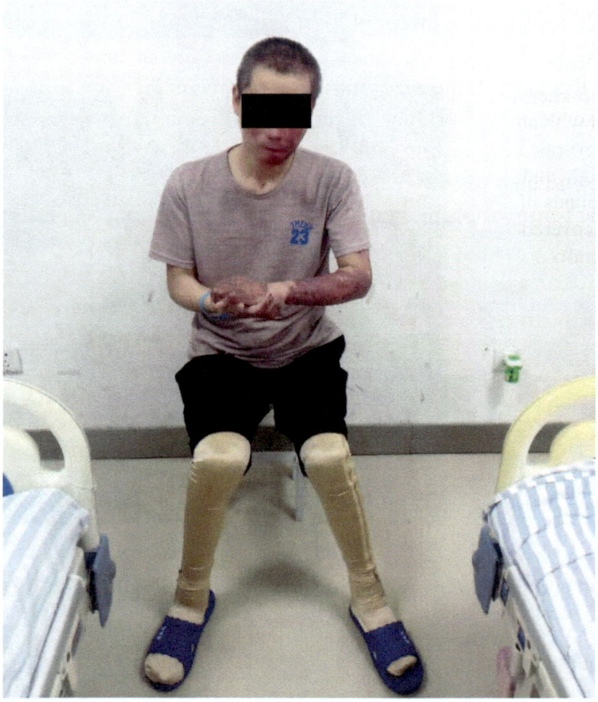

Fig. 3.25 Follow-up at 8 weeks post-injury indicated continued positive progress in both function and appearance of the knee area following rehabilitation exercises

[Discussion]

As the treatment of large and extensive burns constantly advances, it is imperative to prioritize scar prevention from the outset and sustain this approach throughout the entire treatment regimen.

Commonly utilized autografts come in three depths: thin split thickness, thick split thickness, and full thickness. Among them, thick split-thickness grafts containing relatively more dermal tissue are preferred for repairing and reconstructing joint areas post-contracture release due to their elasticity, durability, and reduced propensity for contracture. Precise treatment-wise, the wound-location-specific grafting strategy deploying thick split-thickness autograft sheets to address joint area wounds from the early stage has the following merits:

- Effectively mitigates severe contracture of the joint area
- Reduces the frequency of subsequent scar revision procedures
- Lays foundation for earlier functional exercises
- Promotes a speedy wound healing at mobile joint sites by ensuring secure graft fixation
- Reduces overall surgical time
- Minimizes susceptibility to infection in autografted joint areas

However, several considerations must be kept in mind when implementing this strategy:

- Harvesting depth should never be excessive to jeopardize the donor site's self-healing capacity.
- Should the donor site's self-healing capacity be compromised, back-grafting with its own skin harvests may be necessary.
- Larger skin harvest sizes potentially lead to increased blood loss.
- Hypertrophic scar formation is a potential risk at the donor site.

Central to this strategy is the use of autograft sheets for joint area repair, streamlining wound closure and functional restoration in one step. Practically, if the excised joint area retains a layer of dermal tissue, a thinner sheet may suffice; if fat tissue or fascia is exposed, a perforated, thick, split-thickness autograft sheet is recommended. Key technical points for autograft sheet harvesting include:

- Harvesting a whole sheet almost equivalent in size to the excised joint area's surface area, in uniform thickness
- Perforating the thick split-thickness sheet for optimal drainage
- Minimizing the need for sheet assembly and reducing connections or seams
- Ensuring a healthy granulation base for grafting on wounds with uneven or devitalized fat tissue

In conclusion, implementing the principle of precise treatment and building functional restoration into the management of large and extensive burns from the early stage, the wound-location-specific grafting strategy has the potential to significantly enhance the overall recovery outcomes for burn patients.

(Chuanan Shen, Dongjie Li)

3.3.5 *Enhanced Hemostasis Technique with Elastic Compression for Extremity Excision*

[Background]
Excision, primarily utilized for early removal of necrotic tissue, typically extends to the deep fascial layer in cases of deep burns [46]. Given the potential substantial blood loss in extensive excision, the excision size at one sitting is generally limited to no more than 30% TBSA. The average bleeding volume for every 1% TBSA during excision is reported to be within the range between 100 mL and 150 mL [47–49]. Estimation can be made that the intraoperative bleeding volume might exceed 3000 mL if more than 30% TBSA is excised. Such a degree of blood loss is life-threatening, as a rapid decrease of 30% in the patient's blood volume, which is about 1680 mL in a 70 kg adult, can cause a significant reduction in hemoglobin and effective circulating blood volume, resulting in irreversible ischemia and hypoxia to tissues and organs [50–54]. Should excessive blood loss occur, substantial blood transfusion may be implemented, which introduces risks of complications such as allergic reactions, coagulation disorders, infections, and even hemolysis. Therefore, a strategy to minimize intraoperative blood loss is beneficial to patient stabilization, particularly during large-size excision.

In extensive burn cases, extremity excision typically deploys a tourniquet for blood loss control. And conventionally, the tourniquet is applied to the extremity's root for blood flow block before the initiation of excision. Then there are typically two modalities regarding when to release the tourniquet. The first is to release it right after excision, followed by the grafting procedure. The second is to release it after the completion of grafting and dressing. The first involves several problems. For example, the entire excised area would bleed all at a time upon the release; the vessels would experience reactive dilation due to prior ischemia and hypoxia, and this would further increase bleeding. The second raises concerns such as insufficient hemostasis due to difficulties in identifying small arterial breaks and potential hematomas due to insufficient hemostasis. To address the dilemma, this section introduces a hemostasis technique that utilizes an elastic bandage for "mobile" compression to enhance the performance of tourniquet use during extremity excision.

[Protocol]
Part 1 Extremity excision

1. General anesthesia is administered, followed by the performance of sterilization and draping.
2. Prior to excision, the target extremity is elevated and a roll of elastic bandage is applied, from the far end toward the trunk, to tightly dress the extremity for exsanguination. Then a tourniquet is fixed at the proximal end. After this, the bandage is removed, and excision is performed.

3. During excision, prompt ligation of the breaks of larger vessels and electrocoagulation of smaller ones should be ensured. The total duration of tourniquet application should not exceed 1 h.
4. Excision of deep second-degree wounds should retain viable dermal tissue as much as possible, while that of third-degree wounds should be carried down to the plane of the deep fascial layer.

Part 2 The enhanced hemostasis technique with "mobile" compression

1. Following excision, wound dressing is performed, again from the far end toward the trunk, with 10 cm wide gauze squares that are moistened with epinephrine saline (1:50000). The gauze squares should slightly overlap with each other. After this, an elastic bandage is employed, also from the far end toward the trunk, until the entire surgical area is enwrapped. Upon securement of both the gauze and bandage, the tourniquet can be released.
2. Then the elastic bandage is progressively unwrapped from the upper end, one lap at a time. Meanwhile, the uncovered underlying gauze squares are removed for wound electrocoagulation.
3. After adequate hemostasis of the first lap of wound, bandage release and electrocoagulation are performed for the second lap. This stepwise procedure is performed for the entire surgical field.
4. Then hydrogen peroxide and gentamicin saline are used to rinse the entire wound, after which grafting and compression with sterile dressings are performed. The knee and elbow areas may require small splints to limit mobility. Subsequently, potential exudation and bleeding are carefully monitored.

[Typical Case]
A 31-year-old man suffered burns over his body from a workplace accident which featured hot liquid ejection from a boiler. He received resuscitation, tracheotomy, debridement, dressing changes, and anti-infection therapies at a local healthcare institution. Seven days post-injury, he was transferred to our center.

Admission diagnosis: 90% TBSA burns (deep second-degree, 5%; third-degree, 85%), post-tracheotomy, hypoproteinemia, coagulation disorders, and acid-base imbalance.

Treatment course: On the ninth day post-injury, excision and allografting were performed for the left upper extremity (see Fig. 3.26). At 9:00 am, anesthesia was initiated. At 9:20 am, the trunk end of the extremity received a tourniquet following exsanguination with an elastic bandage. Excision was carried to the fascia for 6% TBSA and finished at 10:04 am. Identified vessel breaks were carefully dealt with by electrocoagulation or ligation. Epinephrine-soaked gauze and dry gauze were used to dress the excised wound. And then an elastic bandage was applied, from the far end toward the trunk, for wound compression. The tourniquet was removed at 10:20 am. The enhanced hemostasis technique was adopted and sufficient hemostasis for the entire surgical area was achieved at 11:05 am. The patient's condition was maintained stable throughout the whole procedure. Following hemostasis, the wound was washed and grafted. The blood-soaked gauze squares were collected to

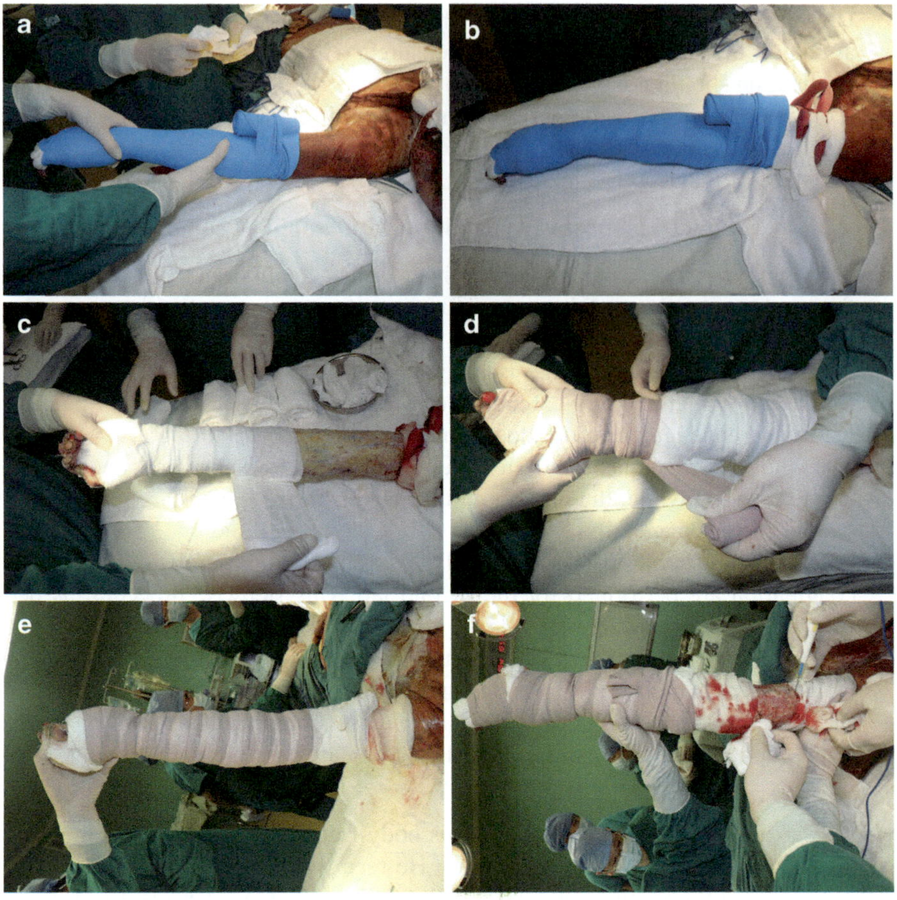

Fig. 3.26 The enhanced hemostasis technique with "mobile" elastic compression. (**a**) Exsanguination. The target extremity is tightly enwrapped, from distal to proximal, with an elastic bandage. (**b**) To block blood flow, a tourniquet is applied to the root area. (**c**) The excised field is enwrapped, from the far end to the trunk, with epinephrine-saline-moistened gauze. (**d**) An elastic bandage is again used, from the far end to the trunk, for compression. (**e**) After adequate compression, the tourniquet is removed. (**f**) The wound was uncovered with section-by-section removal of the bandage and gauze. Electrocoagulation and ligation were performed section by section

calculate the bleeding volume, which turned out to be 318 mL in total. Postoperative inspection revealed no hematoma. Take rate was about 88% on the tenth day post-surgery.

[Discussion]

Burns result in approximately 180,000 fatalities annually worldwide as reported by the World Health Organization [55]. The challenge of repairing extensive burn wounds and saving lives from extensive deep burns remains profound. Before the introduction of early excision and grafting, the primary causes of death in burn patients were infections, invasion into underlying tissue, and even sepsis. The consensus to treat extensive deep burns with early excision and grafting [56] has significantly reduced wound infections and sepsis, shortened hospital stays, lowered patient mortality, and improved cosmetic results and functions [48, 57–59]. It was reported that the early-stage surgical interventions of excision and grafting could reduce mortality from 24% to 7% in adult burn patients [55].

However, the extent of excision at one sitting is seriously limited by blood loss volume. Previous studies have indicated that blood loss for every 1% TBSA during excision can vary considerably, ranging from 77.3 mL, 117 mL, to 170 mL, or even 387 mL [55, 60–63]. Should the excision size exceed 30%, estimated blood loss could escalate to between 2319 and 11,610 mL. Such substantial intraoperative blood loss would precipitate circulatory instability in critical burn patients. As per the grading criteria for shock by Advanced Trauma Life Support, the patient would suffer decompensated shock and irreversible tissue and organ damage when the bleeding volume surpasses 30% of the body's blood volume (that is about 1680 mL in a 70 kg adult) [54]. If that occurs, substantial blood transfusion is demanded for volume return and circulation stability. However, serious complications may ensue, such as infections, hypothermia, coagulation disorders, acid-base imbalance, and systemic inflammatory response syndrome (SIRS). Transfusion has been linked to higher mortality rates in critical burn patients [64–66]. In view of this, a robust hemostasis method to reduce blood loss can be beneficial to patients with extensive burns.

There are two commonly used methods to limit blood loss in critical burn surgeries nowadays. Generally, prior to excision of the trunk and scalp, subcutaneous injection of epinephrine saline is commonly used for bleeding control. The mechanism is the induction of localized vasoconstriction from the injection. As for extremity excision, a tourniquet has been prevalently used. Practically, we found that if the tourniquet is employed for the entire excision, grafting, and dressing process, then, though the intraoperative bleeding volume is controlled, small arterial breaks can be missed during hemostasis. Compression can efficiently manage minor venous bleeding. However, it is less effective for small arteries. Consequently, the patient is more likely to experience hematomas, which compromise the take rate. Alternatively, if we release the tourniquet right after excision and then perform hemostasis and grafting, all the excised areas lose compression and bleed simultaneously. Such a circumstance can be even worse when vessels experience reactive dilatation resulting from ischemia and hypoxia. Since all the bleeding sites cannot be concurrently addressed and the majority are exposed to continuous bleeding, blood loss may become excessive and the operative procedure unstable. This represents the dilemma in tourniquet use nowadays—potential hematomas for release after grafting and compression, and excessive blood loss for release right after excision. With our enhanced hemostasis technique, this dilemma can be properly solved.

Our technique enhances existing compression hemostasis techniques by introducing a "mobile" elastic bandage. The bandage is arranged before tourniquet release for blood flow compression, and after tourniquet release, it is unraveled, lap by lap, to reveal the excised area for sequential hemostasis. This significantly reduces intraoperative blood loss compared with the conventional techniques. The elastic bandage actually serves as a mobile tourniquet, moving proximal-to-distal, and reduces blood loss from the potential bleeding sites queuing for hemostasis. Meanwhile, this stepwise approach also contributes to the reduction in total hemostasis time, further reducing blood loss.

In conclusion, when performing large-size excision, all efforts should converge on a common objective: to reduce operative time, minimize blood loss, and ensure stable patient condition. The enhanced hemostasis technique with elastic compression significantly reduces blood loss and shortens operative time for extremity excision. It is worthy of broader application in the care of patients with extensive burns.

3.4 Meek Grafting to Enable Frequent Harvesting of Autografts from the Same Donor Site on the Trunk or Extremities

[Background]
While advancements have been made in burn care, addressing large or extensive burns remains a complex challenge in clinical practice. A critical factor for successful burn treatment lies in expediting wound closure. Nevertheless, a persistent obstacle in this endeavor has been the scarcity of available autograft donor sites, presenting a significant and enduring challenge that is not easily overcome [67, 68].

The ideal autograft donor site in the management of large or extensive burns should possess properties such as rapid healing, being receptive to frequent harvesting, and minimal scar formation post-healing. These properties are all present in the scalp [69], making it the preferred and primary donor site for patients with significant burns. However, clinically, the scalp's limited size, compounded by the occurrence of deep burns affecting the scalp in a considerable number of patients, presents a formidable challenge. Under such difficult situations, only the donor sites on the trunk, extremities, or buttocks may be available. But these donor sites have several weaknesses [70]:

1. Traditionally, these secondary donor sites allow for only two to three harvesting procedures, after which their surface becomes more fragile, prone to cracking, and susceptible to noticeable scarring.
2. The intervals between successive harvesting sessions are typically lengthy, ranging from 2 to 3 weeks, prolonging the treatment duration and elevating associated risks.
3. Some of these donor sites may develop refractory wounds due to factors like infection and malnutrition, particularly in elderly patients or those with underlying conditions such as diabetes. This directly increases the total wound size, aggravates the patient's condition, and exacerbates the shortage of viable autograft sources.

To strengthen the donor sites on the trunk, extremities, and buttocks, our team has creatively applied Meek autografting [71] to intentionally repair these sites post-harvesting since 2014. With this strategy, we have observed a notable improvement in the healing process of these donor sites, characterized by smoother and accelerated healing, as well as enhanced skin quality upon resurfacing. The reduced intervals between successive harvesting procedures and the overall enhancement in resurfaced skin quality have collectively enabled a heightened frequency of these donor sites, which are thereby transformed into a replenishable autograft reservoir akin to the scalp. Furthermore, the post-healing surfaces of these donor sites following this strategy exhibit diminished scar formation and yield superior cosmetic and functional outcomes.

[Protocol]

I. Indications

1. Patients with large or extensive burns necessitating repeated harvesting from the donor sites on trunk, extremities, or buttocks
2. Geriatric individuals, particularly those with significant comorbidities such as diabetes, requiring extensive skin harvesting from these regions
3. Cases of large or extensive burns where the scalp is not a feasible donor site option

II. Preoperative calculation

The determination of the autograft size to be harvested from these donor sites is contingent upon the surgical method and area. Given that the available autologous skin is at a premium, meticulous preoperative calculations of the surgical area (the size of wounds to be grafted) and the harvest size are imperative. This precision is essential to prevent the need for additional harvesting during surgery or inadvertent waste of autologous skin resources.

After the measurement of the surgical area, the size of autografts needed for burn wound coverage is contingent upon the specific surgical methodology employed. In the context of employing the Meek autografting technique (typically with an expansion ratio of 1:6 or 1:9) to intentionally repair the harvested donor sites, the total size of autografts to be harvested is the sum of that needed for burn wound coverage and that needed for donor site coverage. It is advisable to demarcate the donor sites using a marker to differentiate them from preexisting burn wounds.

III. Perioperative procedure

An appropriate amount of normal saline or epinephrine-containing normal saline (1 μg/ml), depending on the patient's BP, is subcutaneously injected at the donor site. The demarcated areas of the donor sites, either from the trunk, buttocks, or extremities, are harvested with a Zimmer dermatome. Based on the varying depths of the wounds, the harvests generally range from 0.2 to 0.35 mm in thickness and are subsequently made into Meek grafts with an expansion ratio of 1:6 or 1:9.

The donor sites are compressed with gauze soaked in adrenaline-containing normal saline (5 μg/ml) and after adequate hemostasis covered with a portion of the prepared Meek grafts. After appropriate stapling, they are first covered with sulfadiazine silver gauze followed by multiple layers of sterile dressings. Donor sites on the extremities are typically bandaged along with the treatment of the burn wounds, whereas those on the trunk or buttocks may be secured with a belt if necessary.

IV. Postoperative care

Standard postoperative care is given, including anti-infection treatment, dressing changes, and nutritional support, to maintain physiological hemoglobin and albumin levels. The multilayered sterile dressings shall be renewed every 2 to 3 days. Vigilant inspection of the wound is imperative, and noticeable exudation under the gauze should be promptly cleaned. Typically, by the sixth day post-operation, the exudation of the wounds is significantly reduced, and the inner layer of sulfadiazine silver gauze can be kept, upon which Baikerui spray (comprising lysostaphin, lysozyme, chlorhexidine acetate) and human recombinant epidermal growth factor can be applied four times daily. Upon the reepithelialization of the donor sites with the Meek autografts, timely removal of the surface gauze is warranted.

V. Tips

1. The autografts harvested from the donor sites on the trunk, buttocks, or extremities should not be too thick, so as to prevent autograft shrinkage from compromising Meek graft quality.
2. Generally, Vaseline can be utilized for skin lubrication if friction between the dermatome and skin hinders the harvesting procedure. However, it should be noted that if the harvests are intended for Meek graft fabrication, the use of Vaseline should be avoided, for it may impede the adhesion between the autografts and Meek gauze, resulting in the failure of Meek grafting.
3. For donor sites on the trunk, notably in the abdomen lacking bony support for skin fixation, alongside subcutaneous injections to even out and tense the skin surface, an assistant is indispensable to stretch and fortify the skin surrounding the donor site to augment tension at the donor site.
4. Strict hemostasis is required for the harvested donor sites, particularly those that are difficult to press and bandage. Meek grafts are transplanted only after ensuring the absence of active bleeding to prevent potential lifting of the Meek gauze and graft islands by hematomas, which could compromise graft viability.
5. Small splints can be utilized in joint areas such as the knee and elbow to mitigate the impact of joint mobility on graft take.
6. In the absence of infection, the Meek gauze helps preserve the local wound microenvironment, facilitating epithelial cell migration and proliferation. Therefore, it is advisable to retain the gauze during dressing changes until

the graft islands have basically fused. However, the presence of significant exudate accumulation beneath the Meek gauze warrants immediate drainage and removal of contaminated gauze.

7. For donor sites slated for multiple harvesting sessions, it is recommended to avoid excessively thick grafts, opting instead for split-thickness grafts to optimize outcomes.

[Typical Case]

The patient, a 36 -year-old man, sustained extensive flame burns covering 98%TBSA from a diesel tanker explosion. Upon admission to a local emergency department, he underwent procedures including tracheotomy, escharotomies on the trunk and four extremities, and dialysis due to renal failure and persistent anuria. He was transferred to our center 2 days after the accident.

Admission diagnoses: ① Burn size: 98% TBSA, burn depth: 3% TBSA, deep second-degree; 70% TBSA, third-degree; 25% TBSA, fourth-degree. Notably, 2% TBSA of the scalp remained unaffected; ② severe inhalation injury; ③ acute renal failure.

Treatment overview: A series of 17 surgical procedures was conducted to address all burn wounds, alongside a 30-day continuous dialysis regimen to facilitate renal function recovery. Given the extensive burn injuries and limited donor site availability, the healing process of deep second-degree burns on the abdomen was monitored, with potential consideration as an additional donor site to expedite the patient's recovery. Encouragingly, the abdominal donor site exhibited progressive healing and underwent five successive harvesting procedures. To promote rapid healing post-harvesting, a proper portion of Meek grafts with 1:6 expansion ratio was transplanted back to the donor site (referred to as Meek back-grafting). Favorable clinical outcomes were observed, with all donor sites fully healed within a timeframe of 9–11 days. Subsequent follow-up assessments revealed pliable and resilient resurfaced skin with mild scar hypertrophy (Fig. 3.27).

[Discussion]

The scarcity of autograft donor sites presents a significant obstacle in the management of extensive burns. While the scalp is typically preferred for its dense follicular structure, robust vascular supply, and rapid healing capacity for repeated harvesting, challenges arise when patients lack viable scalp tissue. This scenario often necessitates a more complex and prolonged treatment regimen, leading to heightened medical costs and increased mortality risk compared to cases where scalp grafts are available. The main reasons for this are the longer intervals between successive harvests from the same donor site on the trunk, buttocks, or extremities, limited reusability, and a higher risk of nonhealing of these sites, all of which delay overall wound closure and escalate treatment complications. Therefore, a solution is urgently needed to "scalplize" the donor sites from the trunk, buttocks, and extremities, i.e., to increase harvesting frequency from these sites, promoting rapid healing, and transforming them into a replenishable source of autografts.

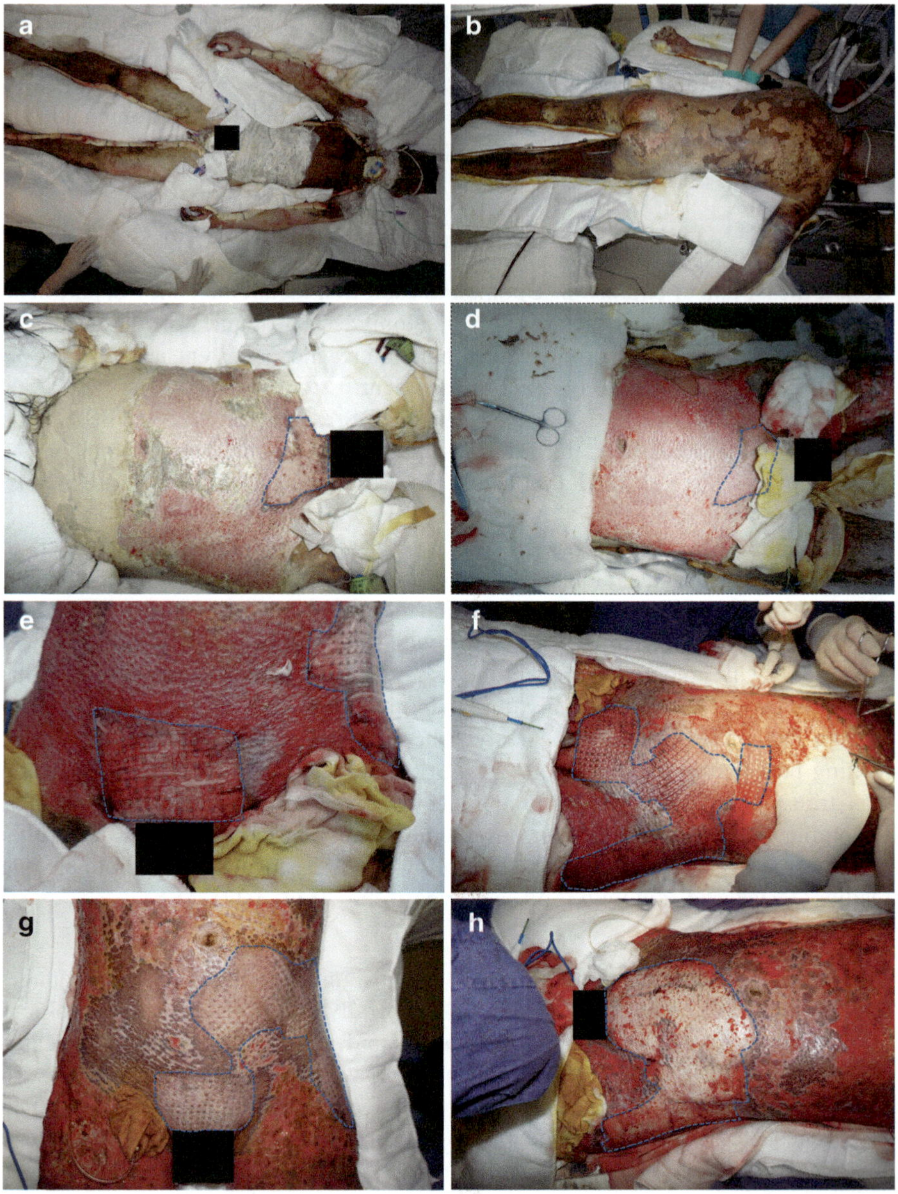

Fig. 3.27 Frequent harvesting of autografts from the same donor site in the abdomen of a patient with 98%TBSA deep burns. (**a**) Anterior view of the patient. The wounds were predominantly third-degree. Escharotomies of the trunk and four extremities had been performed at a local ED. (**b**) Posterior view of the patient. About 2%TBSA of unaffected scalp could be seen, while the rest of the skin all over the body suffered deep burns. (**c**) The first autograft harvesting and Meek back-grafting were performed in the region outlined with the blue dashed line. Obvious maceration of the necrotic tissue on the abdomen was observed. (**d**) The donor site for the first harvesting (outlined with the blue dashed line) healed. The abdominal wounds appeared clean, with no discernible

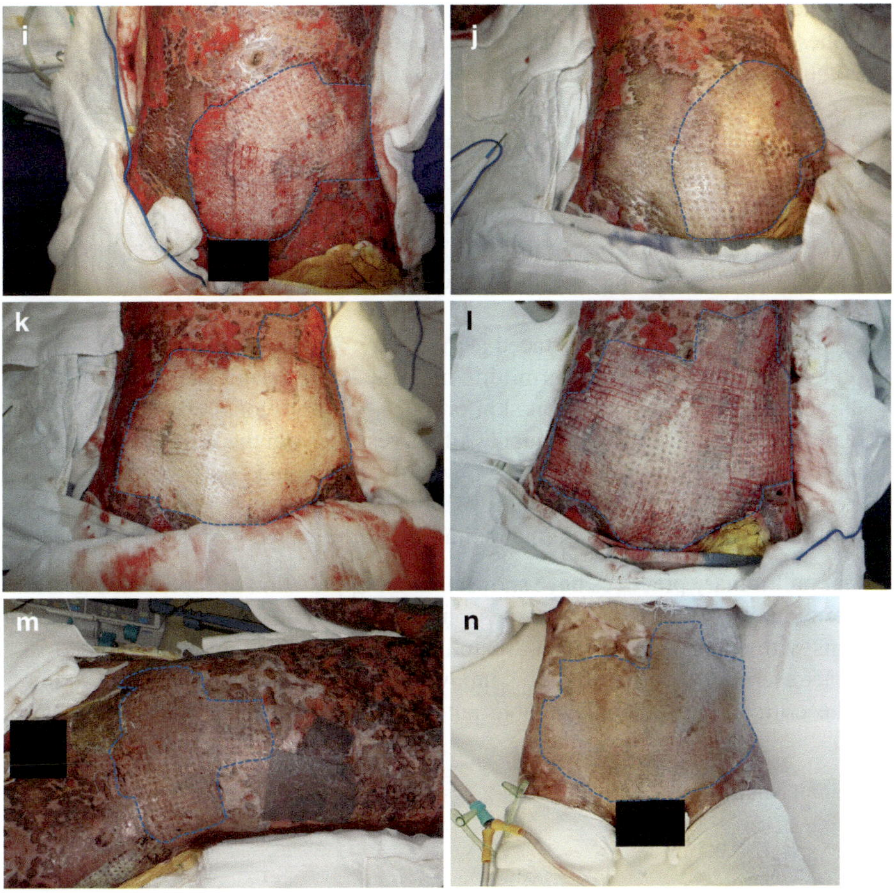

Fig. 3.27 (continued) presence of necrotic tissue adhering to the surface. (**e**) More abdominal wounds achieved healing and could serve as additional donor sites. The second harvesting and Meek back-grafting were performed in regions outlined with blue dashed lines. Healing of the burn wounds was in steady progress. (**f**) The third harvesting and Meek back-grafting were performed in regions outlined with the blue dashed line. The residual unhealed wounds were clean, with noticeable fusion of graft islands. (**g**) The donor sites for the third harvesting (outlined with the blue dashed line) exhibited satisfactory healing outcomes. (**h**) The fourth harvesting was performed in the region outlined with the blue dashed line. (**i**) Meek back-grafting was performed following the fourth harvesting. (**j**) The donor site for the fourth harvesting (outlined with the blue dashed line) healed with satisfactory skin quality. (**k**) The fifth harvesting from an expanded donor site (outlined with the blue dashed line) was performed. (**l**) Meek back-grafting was performed following the fifth harvesting. (**m**) The donor site for the fifth harvesting (outlined with the blue dashed line) healed well. (**n**) Follow-up 1 year later showed that the resurfaced skin at the abdominal donor site (outlined with the blue dashed line) was pliable and resilient, with light scar hyperplasia

To find such a solution, we have tried the transplantation of Meek autografts back onto these donor areas in patients with extensive burns, yielding favorable clinical outcomes. Contrasting traditional approaches, this strategy offers several advantages:

- Enhanced healing rates: Notably, over 200 operations utilizing the new method have demonstrated successful healing outcomes, with only two exceptions of wounds on foot dorsum.
- Expedited healing: Meek grafts with expansion ratios of 1:6 typically achieve complete epithelialization within 8 to 12 days, while those with a 1:9 ratio require 2 to 3 weeks, surpassing the slower healing time, typically 14 ~ 23 days, with conventional methods.
- Significantly improved resurfaced skin quality: The strategy results in durable, pliable skin at donor sites, permitting multiple harvests and surpassing the limitations of thinner, less resilient skin produced by traditional approaches. In our experience, the maximum frequency of harvesting from the same donor site was up to 5 with the new strategy and a 3 with the traditional approach.
- Reduced scarring: The donor sites exhibit minimal scar hyperplasia following treatment, further enhancing their suitability for repeated grafting.

Our preliminary practices have shown that the application of Meek back-grafting to intentionally repair the donor sites on the trunk, buttocks, and extremities in patients with extensive burns can "scalplize" these donor sites, establishing a sustainable reservoir of autografts. This innovative strategy shows promise in addressing the critical shortfall of available autografts for patients with extensive burn injuries.

(Chuanan Shen, Jianhua Cai)

3.5 NPWT with Allograft Cushion to Manage Infected Burn Wound

[Background]
Wound infection constitutes the predominant complication of extensive burns. Generally, such infection can be controlled by local debridement, dressing changes and judicious administration of antibiotics [72, 73]. However, any untimely response has the potential to exacerbate infection, permitting invasion of deeper tissues and structures and even precipitating a life-threatening septic condition if bacteria infiltrate the circulatory system.

Our team has been utilizing a novel approach incorporating "allograft cushion" into negative pressure wound therapy (NPWT) to manage extensive infected burn wounds on extremities, particularly those that are refractory or demonstrate non-healing characteristics. This approach provides both structural support and therapeutic benefits to facilitate granulation growth, thereby creating conducive conditions for subsequent grafting procedures. When implemented with precision and caution, this method yields highly promising clinical outcomes.

[Key Technical Points]

The key technical points of this approach to treating infected burn wounds are as follows:

1. Proper allograft (usually porcine skin) is utilized to provide a circular coverage at the root of the extremity, upon which NPWT sealant films can be securely attached to facilitate a well-sealed environment. The circular coverage is therefore referred to as the "cushion."
2. In the event of substantial necrotic tissue or exudate that cannot be completely debrided at one sitting, the NPWT device could be placed for about 2 ~ 3 days after the first operation, so as to prevent the obstruction of the foam's pores, which could compromise drainage efficiency. A cleaner wound bed may typically accommodate the device for an extended period of 3 ~ 5 days.
3. Excess or viscous drainage content necessitates the use of washout tubing through which nitrofurazone or gentamicin saline solution can be intermittently given for effective wound irrigation.
4. It is of paramount importance to ensure the wound remains sealed, with efficient drainage sustained under negative pressure.
5. It is important to keep alert to the changes in the patient's routine blood tests and body temperature. Bacterial culture is necessary each time the NPWT device is removed or renewed. This enables timely adjustments of antibiotic treatment in accordance with the culture results, thereby optimizing the therapeutic response.

[Typical Case]

The patient, a 37 year-old-man who sustained multiple molten metal burns to the body, was sent to our center 27 h after the accident. On May 20, 2012, the patient experienced an unfortunate accident at his workplace, where he inadvertently slipped and fell into a reservoir containing molten metal. It is estimated that the depth of the metal pool was approximately 0.5 meters, with a temperature between 700 ~ 800 °C. Upon contact, the patient sustained multiple burn injuries and promptly climbed out of the site. He arrived at our center 27 h post-injury.

Admission diagnosis: ① Burn size: 80% TBSA; burn depth: grade III; ② post-tracheotomy.

Physical examination: After an intensive 20-day treatment regimen, the wounds on the trunk and both upper extremities basically healed. However, the wounds on both lower extremities and the buttocks persisted in their nonhealing state attributable to infection caused by extensively drug-resistant *Pseudomonas aeruginosa*. Concurrently, the patient also manifested typical signs of sepsis, such as delirium, a fever reaching 40 °C, a WBC count of 26.5×10^9/L, a neutrophil percentage exceeding 93%, along with a severe lung infection. Despite repeated debridement and daily dressing changes, the wounds remained refractory to healing. Additionally, the graft take of multiple grafting procedures was notably low (Fig. 3.28).

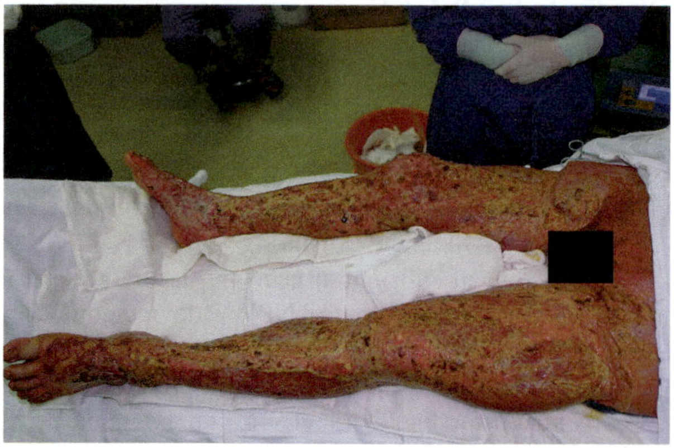

Fig. 3.28 Infection of wounds on both lower extremities

Treatment Overview

1. General treatment protocol

   - Resuscitation and anti-shock treatment.
   - A two-pronged nutritional support, both enterally and parenterally, to strengthen nutrition supply.
   - Blood sugar control.
   - Specific medications were administered to safeguard the functionality of vital organs.
   - Dynamic administration of antibiotics based on experience and subsequent results of bacterial culture. Upon admission, the patient was initially administered a combination of imipenem and vancomycin, based on our experience. However, bacterial culture results dated May 30 revealed the presence of *Pseudomonas aeruginosa* which was sensitive to piperacillin, and *Acinetobacter baumannii* which was sensitive to levofloxacin. Consequently, the antibiotic regimen was accordingly modified to include piperacillin and levofloxacin and preserve the use of vancomycin to prevent staphylococcal infections. The initial imipenem course was discontinued, and caspofungin was introduced as a prophylactic measure against potential fungal infection.
   - Gamma globulin and thymosin were given to boost immunity.
   - Psychological counseling.

2. Wound management protocol

   Following the initial debridement of the wounds on both lower extremities, NPWT was performed in combination with intermittent washout of the wounds and intermittent flow of pure oxygen to the sub-atmospheric space (Figs. 3.29 and 3.30). The NPWT dressings were removed on the third postoperative day. Notably, the dressings exhibited conspicuous green stains, localizing to areas overlaid by necrotic tissue. The rest of the wounds appeared cleaner with an overall improvement in their condition (Figs. 3.31 and 3.32). Subsequently, the second surgical debridement was performed.

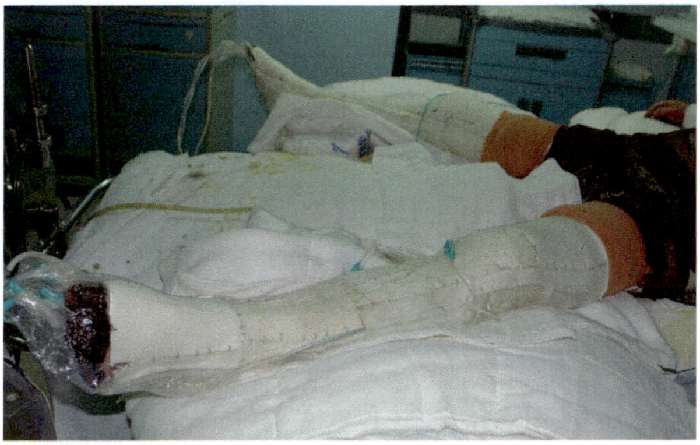

Fig. 3.29 Application of NPWT to refractory infected burn wounds. After debridement, the wounds were treated with NPWT dressings, which were connected to continuous negative pressure and suction devices, in combination with wound irrigation and oxygen delivery through tubing placed inside the dressings

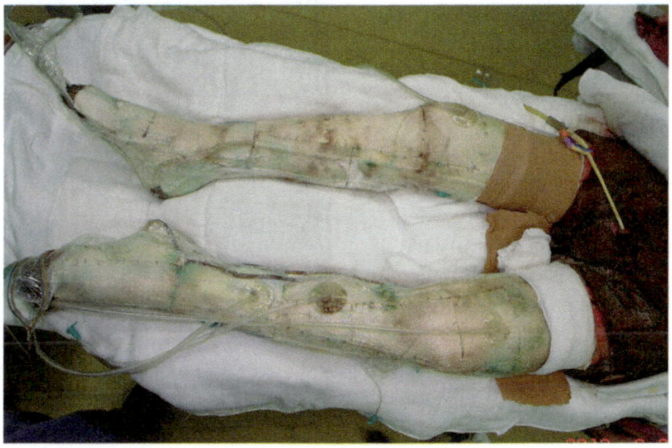

Fig. 3.30 On the third day following the first operation, the NPWT dressings displayed sporadic patches of green staining

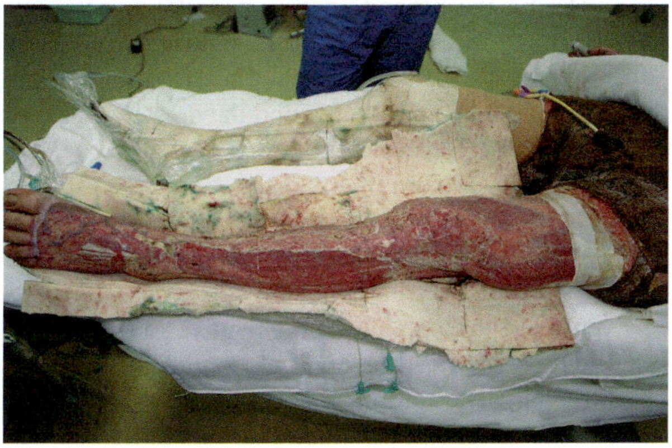

Fig. 3.31 Based on the aforementioned observations, the NPWT was removed from the left lower extremity. It was discerned that the patches of green staining corresponded to wound areas overlaid by necrotic tissue. However, the rest of the wounds appeared clean, and the dressings applied over these areas exhibited no evidence of green staining

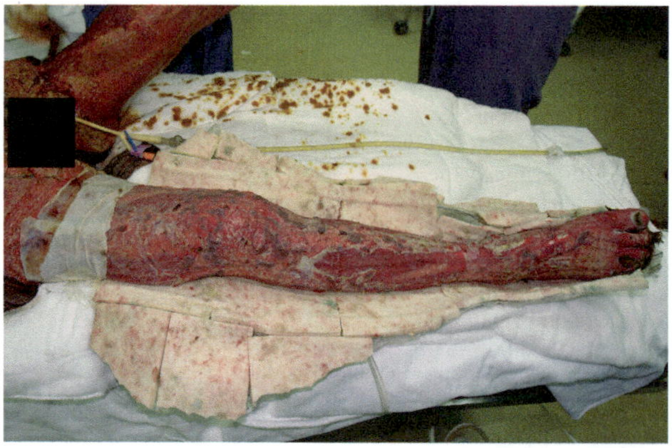

Fig. 3.32 NPWT dressings and wound conditions on the right extremity mirrored those observed on the left

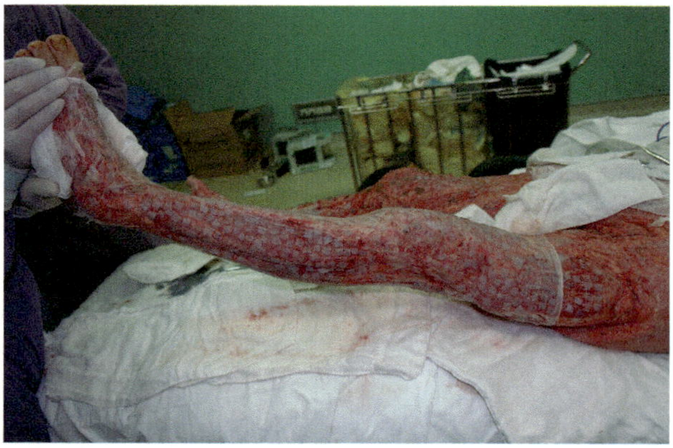

Fig. 3.33 The second operation was performed, during which debridement was repeated, and intermingled transplantation of a small quantity of autografts and donor skin grafts provided by the patient's family to the wounds on both lower extremities was performed

During the second operation, following the intermingled transplantation of autografts and allografts from family donation to the wounds on both lower extremities (Fig. 3.33), continuous NPWT was conducted. The NPWT dressings were removed 3 days later, and the dressings also exhibited obvious green stains (Fig. 3.34). However, the grafts were in place and the wounds were comparatively clean, devoid of any discernible green staining (Fig. 3.35).

This pattern of debridement coupled with continuous NPWT was repeated several times. As the wounds progressively improved, the interval for NPWT replacement was incrementally extended. These concerted efforts effectively controlled the patient's wound infection and fresh granulation formed on the wound bed, creating optimal conditions for grafting (Figs. 3.36 and 3.37). Subsequently, multiple grafting procedures were performed to close the wounds (Fig. 3.38). The patient was eventually extricated from the dangerous condition.

3. Follow-up observations

   Upon subsequent follow-up, all wounds had completely healed. After a period of rehabilitative exercises, the functional outcomes of both lower extremities were deemed satisfactory.

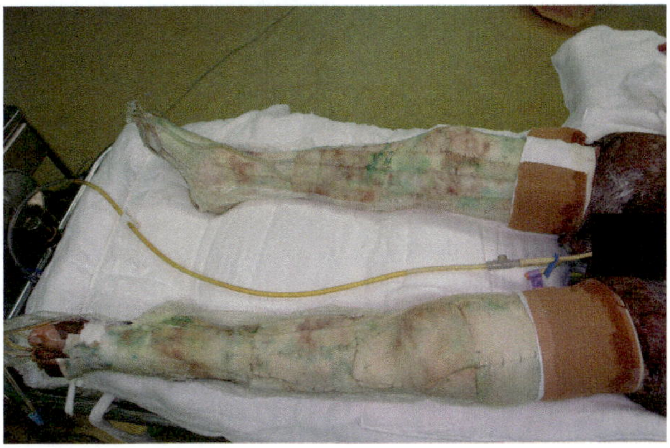

Fig. 3.34 On the third day following the second operation, patches of green staining were also noted on the dressings

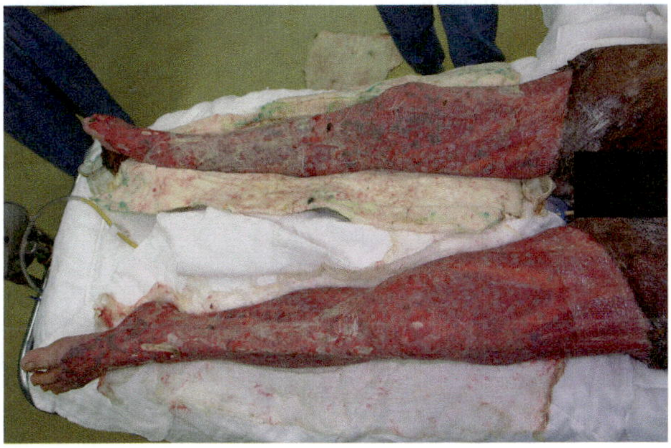

Fig. 3.35 Upon removal of the dressings, despite the presence of green stains, it was noted that the grafts remained in place, and the wound surfaces were relatively clean

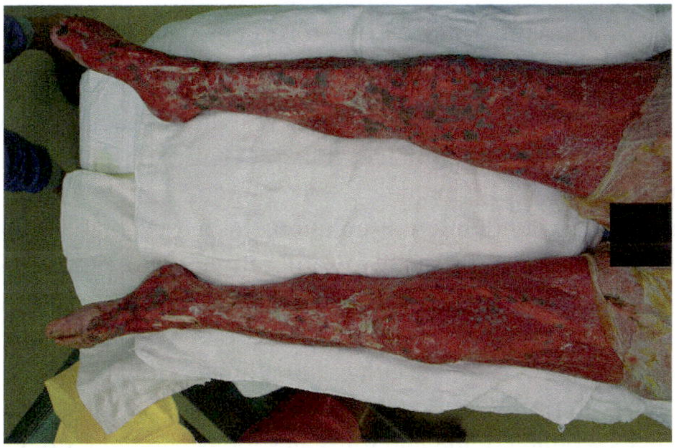

Fig. 3.36 Wound condition during the third operation. NPWT was continued after grafting

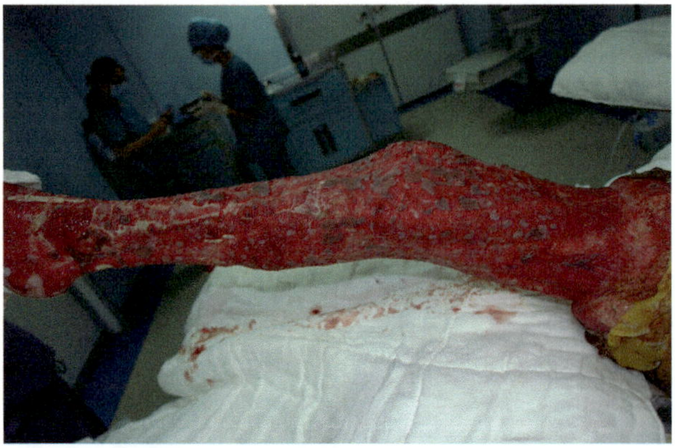

Fig. 3.37 One week following the third operation, the NPWT dressings were removed, fresh granulation was observed, and the graft rake was deemed satisfactory. After an additional two procedures involving debridement and grafting, the wounds eventually achieved complete healing

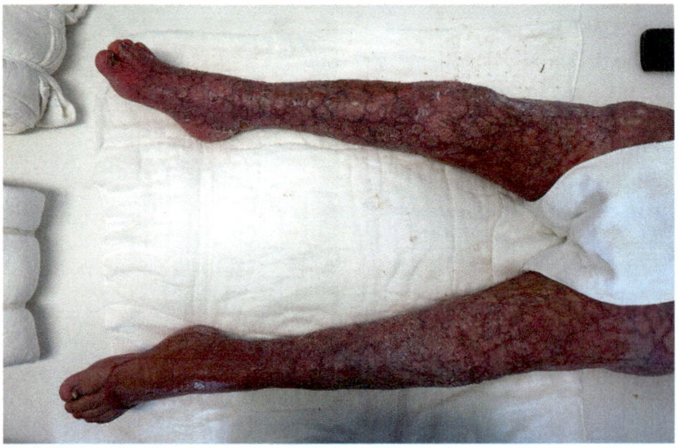

Fig. 3.38 Conditions of both lower extremities upon complete wound healing

[Discussion]

The advantages of applying NPWT to burn wounds can be summarized as follows [74–81]:

- The full and tight contact between the NPWT dressings and the wound surface facilitates optimal exudate drainage, thus preventing infections that could arise from the accumulation of exudate.
- NPWT improves wound microcirculation, increases the capillary density in acute wounds, stimulates fibroblast proliferation, and encourages angiogenesis and granulation growth. These factors collectively expedite wound healing.
- NPWT also increase the expression and release of various pertinent growth factors and enzymes, such as vascular endothelial growth factor and fibroblast growth factor-2, to promote reepithelialization.
- NPWT reduces wound edema and mitigates the detrimental effects of inflammatory mediators, lactic acid, and other substances in exudate, forming a favorable environment to promote wound healing.

For cases without healthy skin around the wound with which to secure the transparent adhesive sealant film, we have introduced the “allograft cushion” method.

This technique utilizes commercially available allogeneic dermis as a cushion, which is affixed to the adjacent eschar or granulation tissue. It is properly dried with a dryer and affixed with skin staples to ensure firm adherence. Subsequently, the NPWT sealant film is applied to the dried allograft, creating an airtight negative pressure environment.

(Shen Chuan'an, Li Dawei)

3.6 An Integrated Approach to Dressing Change

3.6.1 Dressing Changes with Considerations of Wound Locations, Wound Types, Treatment Time, and Temperature

[Background]
Dressing change, a basic skill involved in wound care, aims to create a favorable environment by removing exudate and necrotic tissue to either encourage epithelialization for wound healing or promote granulation growth for grafting. For wounds that share similar conditions, different dressing approaches may yield markedly disparate outcomes [82, 83]. Conversely, a standard and proper strategy of dressing change can greatly reduce the risk of wound infection and enhance the overall patient outcome [11]

From our experience, we have concluded an integrated approach to dressing change that coordinates three main aspects concerned with this process: locations of wounds, cleanliness of different wounds, and optimization of dressing change scheduling. Considerations of the three aspects are helpful to prevent excessive wound exposure, delineate procedural priorities, and ensure enough rest for the patient [12]. Additionally, the approach also emphasizes the importance of monitoring the temperature of solutions involved in the procedures to secure optimal sterilization and irrigation results [84].

[Protocol]

I. Sequential treatment for multiple affected body regions

Extensive burns often involve various body regions simultaneously, including the trunk, extremities, scalp, face, and perineum. Consideration of the affected areas emphasizes that dressings on the extremities and trunk should not be simultaneously removed to avoid unnecessary exposure, which heightens the risk of bacterial colonization and subsequent infection [85]. Instead, wounds in different areas should be attended to in a specified sequence. Different regions, namely the scalp and face, anterior trunk, posterior trunk, extremities, perineum, and incision areas of tracheotomy, deep venous or arterial catheterization, should be treated one by one sequentially. Separate care kits and dressings should be prepared for each region to prevent cross-infection, and disposable gloves should be replaced between treatments of different areas.

II. Differentiated treatments for clean and contaminated wounds
Differentiated plans should be tailored to treat wounds varying in cleanliness. Wounds with a clean surface can be dressed and bandaged every other day. Contaminated or infected wounds necessitate more thorough debridement and more frequent dressing changes to promote the removal of necrotic tissue and the drainage of exudate [86]. Wounds of varying cleanliness should also be bandaged separately, so as to facilitate localized, differentiated treatment and prevent cross-contamination [87].
III. Optimized timing for dressing change
Dressing changes are typically scheduled for the morning hours to allow the patient an uninterrupted rest period at noon. For localized wounds that are infected and require an additional dressing change, the procedure should be added in the afternoon or evening.
IV. Appropriate temperature for involved solutions
A thermostatic water bath is employed to preheat the iodophor and normal saline to a temperature of 40 °C and the enzymatic disinfectants (such as lysozyme) to 37 °C before application. During dressing changes, it is essential to maintain the patient's warmth.

[Typical Case]

The patient, a 70-year-old male, presented with multiple flame burns sustained during an incident of burning weeds in the wild, during which he caught fire and subsequently rolled into a nearby stream. He was initially discovered by passerby and transported to a local hospital within his county, where he received fluid resuscitation and debridement. Subsequently, he was referred to a superior medical facility in the capital city of his province. Two days post-referral, he underwent a tracheotomy, skin harvesting from the abdomen, and grafting for the neck area. Twelve days post-procedure, he was transferred to our center. Upon admission, he was conscious but exhibited symptoms of oliguria, sleep deprivation, lack of appetite, and poor nutritional status.

Past medical history: A 18-year history of diabetes, two episodes of stroke 7 years prior, hypertension for over a year (160/70 mmHg), and 8-month history of chest tightness and shortness of breath (diagnosed with coronary heart disease at a local medical facility).

Specialized physical examination: Burn wounds were identified on the patient's head, face, neck, wrists, lower extremities, buttocks, posterior trunk, and other areas, with a total burn size of about 60% TBSA (Fig. 3.39). A significant amount of purulent exudate was present on the face and neck, and other wounds were covered by eschars, beneath which pus was evident. An autograft measuring approximately 5 cm × 12 cm could be observed on the neck with poor graft take. Tracheotomy had been performed with successful placement and functioning of the tube. Aspiration revealed a large amount of sputum. The wounds on both lower extremities, buttocks, and posterior trunk exhibited a charred appearance, with some showing accumulation of pus under the eschar and loss of tenderness. Some wounds on both lower extremities presented as erythematous and pallid. An unhealed donor site measuring approximately 1% TBSA was identified on the left lower abdomen. Peripheral blood supply was satisfactory.

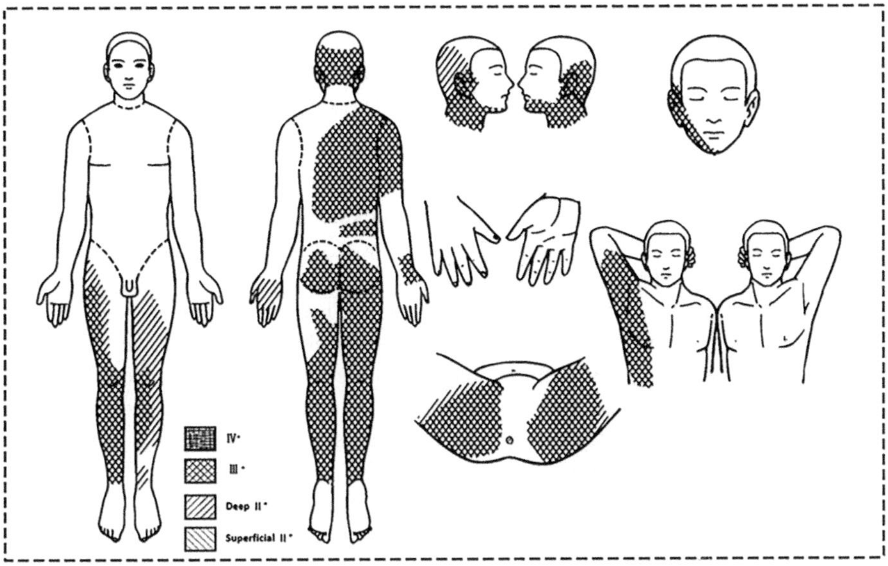

Surface Area (Rule of Nines)

		TBSA%
Head &Neck	Scalp	3
	Face	3
	Neck	3
Trunk	Anterior trunk	13
	Posterior trunk	13
	Perineum	1
Upper extremities	Upper arms	7
	Lower arms	6
	Hands	5
Lower extremities	Buttocks	5
	Thighs	21
	Legs	13
	Feet	7
	Total	100

Relative Burn Size

	Superficial II°	Deep II°	III°	IV°
Scalp		1	1	
Face		2	1	
Neck			2	
Anterior trunk				
Posterior trunk		1	12	
Perineum				
Upper arms			4	
Lower arms				
Hands		1		
Buttocks			4	
Thighs		4	15	
Legs		1	11	
Feet				
Total		10	50	
Burn Size	60% TBSA			

Fig. 3.39 Burn profile of the 70-year-old male patient

Admission diagnoses: ① Burn size: 60% TBSA; deep second-degree, 10% TBSA; third-degree, 50% TBSA; burns to multiple body parts; ② inhalation injury, tracheotomy, bilateral pneumonia; ③ wound infection; ④ anemia; ⑤ hypoproteinemia; ⑥ diabetes; ⑦ hypertension (grade 2); ⑧ coronary heart disease; ⑨ sequelae of stroke.

Treatment Overview

For the third-degree wounds on the back, buttocks, right upper arm, and both legs, 1% iodine tincture was applied, and a dryer was continuously used to facilitate eschar desiccation. The remaining wounds were categorized into three groups: both hands, both thighs, and the head, face, and neck. The three groups were addressed sequentially. Treatment commenced with the bilateral hands, which were comparatively clean, proceeded to the thighs, and concluded with the head, face, and neck. The latter region displayed a higher degree of contamination, characterized by an excess of purulent exudates and positive cultures for *Pseudomonas aeruginosa*, thereby demanding meticulous attention and care.

Dressing changes were primarily scheduled for the morning hours. For the face and neck areas, an additional brief debridement in the afternoon was performed, and a renewal of the dressing materials was flexibly arranged in the night, depending on the exudate levels and the patient's body temperature. Prior to each procedure, iodophor and normal saline solutions were preheated in a thermostatic water bath to a temperature of 40 °C. During the morning dressing change, gauze pads soaked in these solutions were used to gently dab and clean the exudate and necrotic tissue from the wounds. This process was repeated several times until a satisfactory result was achieved. Direct irrigation was avoided.

With this approach, the exudate on the face and neck areas gradually decreased, residual eschars dissolved, and granulation tissue proliferated. Two weeks post-admission, bacterial culture results for the facial and neck wounds turned negative, with no positive cultures for *Pseudomonas aeruginosa* in other wounds. Three weeks post-admission, face and neck debridement, harvest from the trunk, and autografting were performed to close the wound. For the wounds on the lower extremities, back, and buttocks, eschar excision and grafting were performed on the 4th, 11th, and 15th days post-admission. All wounds were closed and eventually healed.

[Discussion]

The concept underpinning this integrated approach to dressing changes is straightforward, akin to addressing a single oil droplet on a table surface. If one indiscriminately cleans the entire table, the solitary oil droplet will spread across the surface, transforming a simple task into a more complex one—cleaning an entire layer of oil film, which is decidedly more arduous and time-consuming. Alternatively, cleaning the uncontaminated surrounding area first, followed by the oil spot, yields a more efficient outcome [88]. This analogy is applicable to the process of changing dressings on burn wounds.

Likewise, the efficacy of oil stain removal varies when using warm water compared to cold. In the context of dressing changes, disinfectants at 39–40 °C are most effective for wound cleaning. Certain enzymatic products exhibit bactericidal properties, functioning optimally at approximately 37 °C [89]. Deviation from this temperature, either higher or lower, can diminish enzyme activity. Therefore, pre-heating of disinfectants and enzymatic products is advised. Furthermore, the warmed solution not only reduces discomfort but also prevents body temperature loss and energy consumption.

(Shen Chuan'an, Sun Tianjun)

3.6.2 *Dynamic Management*

[Background]
The wound repair of patients with large burns is a dynamic process [90]. As the treatment progresses, the shallow wounds gradually heal, while the deeper wounds are repaired through skin grafting [91].The actual total wound size is constantly changing during the course of treatment. Correspondingly, the patient's fluid requirements, metabolic needs, and nutritional supplementation must be continuously adjusted to meet the evolving clinical scenario. The initial burn area assessment at the time of diagnosis may no longer accurately reflect the actual wound status. Therefore, the authors propose a new dynamic management strategy for large-area burn wounds [92]. At 2, 3, 4, and 5 weeks post-burn, the wound types are reevaluated and categorized; the size of different types of wounds is reassessed, and the corresponding nutritional needs are dynamically estimated. This approach can guide the formulation of precise, stage-appropriate treatment measures throughout the patient's recovery.

[Protocol]

I. Dynamic assessment of wound types and size to facilitate stage-appropriate wound care strategies

   1. The wound assessment graph is utilized to evaluate the burn sizes and depths of different wounds in the early post-burn period. The sizes of superficial second-degree, deep second-degree, third-degree, and fourth-degree wounds should be specified [93].
   2. The wound types and sizes are dynamically evaluated at 2, 3, 4, and 5 weeks post-burn. The evaluation includes the initial wound size, the healed size, the operated yet unhealed size, the size of the wounds to be grafted (these wounds can be covered with biological dressings, eschar, or granulation bed), and the size of wounds that could be healed with dressing changes. The wounds were given dynamic treatment based on their changing types and sizes (Table 3.3) [94].

II. Dynamic calculation of wound size and nutritional needs

   Nutrition and fluid requirements are calculated along with the dynamic calculation of wound size, which excludes the healed wounds and those covered with allograft [95].

Table 3.3 Dynamic evaluation of burn wound

Body part	Initial burn size	Healed size	Operated yet unhealed size	Wounds awaiting grafting			Wounds that could be healed with dressing changes
				With biological dressing	With eschar coverage	With granulation	
Head 3%							
Face 3%							
Neck 3%							
Trunk 27%							
Upper arms 7%							
Forearms 6%							
Hands 5%							
Buttocks 5%							
Thighs 21%							
Lower legs 13%							
Feet 7%							
Total 100%							

[Typical Case]

The patient, a 51-year-old man, sustained multiple burns caused by an LPG explosion and was admitted to a hospital 5 hours post-burn. There was no history of coma, but he presented with hoarseness and expectoration, for which tracheotomy was performed.

Past medical history: Hypertension, diabetes, and cerebral infarction.

Admission diagnoses: ① Total burn size, 92%; superficial second-degree, 2%; deep second-degree, 20%; third-degree, 70% (Fig. 3.40); ② inhalation injury; ③ post-tracheotomy.

Dynamic Wound Management

1. **Wound evaluation 2 weeks post-burn**

On the third post-burn day, the patient underwent excision of the left upper limb and right lower limb (limb grouping I), Meek grafting, xenograft coverage, and autograft harvesting from the head and anterior trunk.

On the fifth day after injury, excision of the right upper limb and left lower limb (limb grouping II), Meek grafting, xenograft coverage, and autograft harvesting from the right upper limb, left lower limb, and anterior trunk were performed. Two weeks after the injury, the four limbs all underwent excision and grafting. The wounds on the trunk and buttocks were covered with eschars, for which the

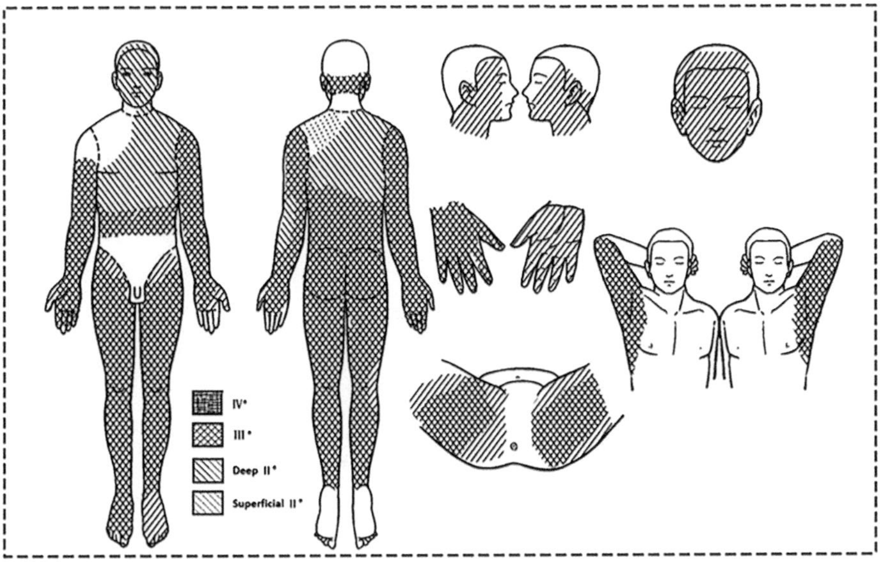

Surface Area (Rule of Nines)

		TBSA%
Head &Neck	Scalp	3
	Face	3
	Neck	3
Trunk	Anterior trunk	13
	Posterior trunk	13
	Perineum	1
Upper extremities	Upper arms	7
	Lower arms	6
	Hands	5
Lower extremities	Buttocks	5
	Thighs	21
	Legs	13
	Feet	7
	Total	100

Relative Burn Size

	Superficial II°	Deep II°	III°	IV°
Scalp		1		
Face		3		
Neck		3		
Anterior trunk		6	5	
Posterior trunk	2	5	7	
Perineum				
Upper Arms			6	
Lower arms			6	
Hands		1	4	
Buttocks			5	
Thighs			21	
Legs			13	
Feet		1	3	
Total	2	20	70	
Burn size	92% TBSA			

Fig. 3.40 Burn profile of the 51-year-old patient

Table 3.4 Dynamic evaluation of burn wounds (2 weeks post-burn)

Body part	Initial burn size	Healed size	Operated yet unhealed size	Wounds awaiting grafting			Wounds that could be healed with dressing changes
				With biological dressing	With eschar coverage	With granulation	
Head 3%	1					1	
Face 3%	3					3	
Neck 3%	3					3	
Trunk 27%	25	2	2		21		
Upper arms 7%	6		5		1		
Forearms 6%	6		6				
Hands 5%	5		2		3		
Buttocks 5%	5				5		
Thighs 21%	21		11	5	5		
Lower legs 13%	13		11	2			
Feet 7%	4		4				
Total 100%	92	2	41	7	35	7	

application of 1% iodine tincture was continued. The debridement and dressing changes for the head, face, and neck wounds were also continued (Table 3.4).

2. **Wound evaluation 3 weeks post-burn**

On the 19th post-burn day, the posterior trunk and buttocks received excision and Meek grafting. Autograft harvesting was performed on the head and posterior trunk. The two limb groupings were treated sequentially, with the outer dressings being replaced. Three weeks after the injury, the wounds on the head, face, and neck healed. The anterior trunk experienced macerating eschar and received debridement and dressing changes. Dressing changes were performed for the two limb groupings on an alternate day basis (Table 3.5).

3. **Wound evaluation 4 weeks post-burn**

Four weeks after injury, the anterior trunk and right lower limb received debridement, Meek grafting, postage-stamp skin grafting, and the head and anterior trunk underwent excision.

Table 3.5 Dynamic evaluation of burn wounds (3 weeks post-burn)

Body part	Initial burn size	Healed size	Operated yet unhealed size	Wounds awaiting grafting			Wounds that could be healed with dressing changes
				With biological dressing	With eschar coverage	With granulation	
Head 3%	1					1	
Face 3%	3	3					
Neck 3%	3	3					
Trunk 27%	25	3	13		9		
Upper arms 7%	6	1	5				
Forearms 6%	6		6				
Hands 5%	5		2		3		
Buttocks 5%	5		5				
Thighs 21%	21		11	5	5		
Lower legs 13%	13		11	2			
Feet 7%	4		4				
Total 100%	92	10	57	7	17	1	

Certain amount of eschars remained at the root of the lateral side of the right thigh. Both hands had eschars and scattered wounds. Wounds on both upper limbs basically healed with reepithelialization of the Meek grafts. The left lower limb was observed with healing and limited residual wounds (Table 3.6).

4. **Wound evaluation 5 weeks post-burn**

Five weeks after the injury, the wounds on the posterior trunk and hip had healed, the anterior trunk had undergone Meek grafting and postage-stamp skin grafting, the right lower limb had undergone postage-stamp skin grafting, and the residual wounds were located at the dorsum of the hands and fingers, the root of the left lower limb, and the right thigh. Subsequently, the wounds underwent two surgical debridements, postage-stamp autograft grafting, and eventually healed (Table 3.7).

[Discussion]

In the course of treatment, the constant changes of the total burn size and wound types dictate alterations of the treatment strategy [96]. Particularly, the exposed wounds, with increased water evaporation, nutritional consumption, and higher risk of infection, require careful evaluation and care [97, 98]. A dynamic evaluation of the wound size in stages is essential for implementing precise burn treatment [99].

(Shen Chuan'an, Sun Tianjun)

Table 3.6 Dynamic evaluation of burn wound (4 weeks post-burn)

Body part	Initial burn size	Healed size	Operated yet unhealed size	Wounds awaiting grafting: With biological dressing	With eschar coverage	With granulation	Wounds that could be healed with dressing changes
Head 3%	1	1					
Face 3%	3	3					
Neck 3%	3	3					
Trunk 27%	25	3	22				
Upper arms 7%	6	5	1				
Forearms 6%	6	6					
Hands 5%	5	3	1		1		
Buttocks 5%	5		5				
Thighs 21%	21	11	9		1		
Lower legs 13%	13	9	4				
Feet 7%	4		4				
Total 100%	92	44	46		2		

Table 3.7 Dynamic evaluation of burn wound (5 weeks post-burn)

Body part	Initial burn size	Healed size	Operated yet unhealed size	Wounds awaiting grafting: With biological dressing	With eschar coverage	With granulation	Wounds that could be healed with dressing changes
Head 3%	1	1					
Face 3%	3	3					
Neck 3%	3	3					
Trunk 27%	25	16	9				
Upper arms 7%	6	6					
Forearms 6%	6	6					
Hands 5%	5	3	2				
Buttocks 5%	5	5					
Thighs 21%	21	16	5				
Lower legs 13%	13	11	2				
Feet 7%	4	4					
Total 100%	92	74	18				

References

1. Ji C, et al. Mixed grafting of small auto- and cryopreserved Allo-skin for residual wound repair in severe burn patients: a retrospective study. Burns. 2025;51(2):107356.
2. Rafieezadeh D, Abbaspour M. Safety and effectiveness of micropigmentation skin grafting using the Meek method. Int J Burns Trauma. 2024;14(6):107–14.
3. Yin K, et al. A novel combination of keratinocyte and autologous microskin grafting to repair full-thickness skin loss. Eur Surg Res. 2022;63(4):269–77.
4. McGovern KP, Rizzo JA. Major burn injury successfully treated with cultured epithelial autografts, a case series presentation: establishing standard clinical practices. J Burn Care Res. 2023;44(3):709–14.
5. Nagano H, et al. Skin graft with dermis and appendages generated in vivo by cell competition. Nat Commun. 2024;15(1):3366.
6. Chen L, et al. Multicenter effect analysis of one-step acellular dermis combined with autologous ultra-thin split thickness skin composite transplantation in treating burn and traumatic wounds. Int Wound J. 2024;21(1):e14341.
7. Tsiklin IL, et al. In vivo bone tissue engineering strategies: advances and prospects. Polymers (Basel). 2022;14(15)
8. Jorgensen AM, et al. Multicellular bioprinted skin facilitates human-like skin architecture in vivo. Sci Transl Med. 2023;15(716):eadf7547.
9. Chai RJ, Wong WL, Beh CW. Developing a bioink for single-step deposition and maturation of human epidermis. Int J Bioprint. 2023;9(4):738.
10. Cao YL, Liu ZC, Chen XL. Efficacy of hydrosurgical excision combined with skin grafting in the treatment of deep partial-thickness and full-thickness burns: a two-year retrospective study. Burns. 2023;49(5):1087–95.
11. Liu HF, Zhang F, Lineaweaver WC. History and advancement of burn treatments. Ann Plast Surg. 2017;78(2 Suppl 1):S2–8.
12. Jackson D. A clinical study of the use of skin homografts for burns. Br J Plast Surg. 1954;7(1):26–43.
13. Chih-Chun Y, et al. Combined use of cutaneous homografts and autografts in extensive burns. Mowlem-Jackson's phenomenon (author's transl). J Chir (Paris). 1980;117(8–9):443–6.
14. Luo B, et al. Non-myeloablative mixed chimerism approaches and tolerance, a split decision. Eur J Immunol. 2007;37(5):1233–42.
15. Hufnagel B, Ninnemann JL, Hettich R. Immunology of intermingled skin grafts in rats: preliminary results. Burns Incl Therm Inj. 1989;15(1):31–5.
16. Shizhao J, et al. Short- and long-term outcomes of small auto- and cryopreserved allograft skin grafting in those with >60%TBSA deep burn wounds. Burns. 2017;43(1):206–14.
17. Shen C, et al. A novel skin grafting modality: prefabricated large sheet of postage-stamp autografts and allografts to repair extensive burn wounds; a prospective matched-control study. Int J Surg. 2023;109(12):3967–73.
18. Zuo KJ, Medina A, Tredget EE. Important developments in burn care. Plast Reconstr Surg. 2017;139(1):120e–38e.
19. Akita S, et al. Novel application of cultured epithelial autografts (CEA) with expanded mesh skin grafting over an artificial dermis or dermal wound bed preparation. Int J Mol Sci. 2017;19(1)
20. Still JJ, Orlet HK, Law EJ. Use of cultured epidermal autografts in the treatment of large burns. Burns. 1994;20(6):539–41.
21. Fabre JW. Epidermal allografts. Immunol Lett. 1991 Jul;29(1–2):161–5. https://doi.org/10.1016/0165-2478(91)90220-5.
22. Pianigiani E, Ierardi F, Cherubini Di Simplicio F, Andreassi A. Skin bank organization. Clin Dermatol. 2005;23(4):353–6. https://doi.org/10.1016/j.clindermatol.2004.07.016.
23. Jeschke MG, Herndon DN. Burns in children: standard and new treatments. Lancet. 2014;383(9923):1168–78. https://doi.org/10.1016/S0140-6736(13)61093-4.

24. Burd A, Lam PK, Lau H. Allogenic skin: transplant or dressing? Burns. 2002;28(4):358–66. https://doi.org/10.1016/s0305-4179(02)00025-6.
25. Shen C, Deng H, Sun T, Cai J, Li D, Li L, He L, Zhang B, Li D, Wang L, Niu Y. Use of fresh scalp allografts from living relatives for extensive deep burns in children: a clinical study over 7 years. J Burn Care Res. 2021;42(2):323–30. https://doi.org/10.1093/jbcr/iraa155.
26. Shen C, Liu X, et al. An innovated elastic compression hemostasis technique for extremity excision in patients with extensive burns: a prospective clinical randomized controlled trial. Surgery. 2023;173(6):1513–7. https://doi.org/10.1016/j.surg.2023.03.002.
27. Luo G, Fan H, Sun W, et al. Blood loss during extensive escharectomy and auto-microskin grafting in adult male major burn patients. Burns. 2011;37(5):790–3. https://doi.org/10.1016/j.burns.2011.01.021. Epub 2011 Feb 26
28. Wardhana A, Aurino L, Menna C. Preoperative blood loss prediction formulas in burn surgeries: a review. J Burn Care Res. 2023;44(3):641–8. https://doi.org/10.1093/jbcr/irac109.
29. Han ZX. A variety of microorganism species at the burn ward. Zhonghua Wai Ke Za Zhi. 1989;27(9):546–74.
30. Guo Z, Sheng Z, Gao W. Escharectomy during burn shock stage contributed to controlling or alleviating infectious complication. Zhonghua Wai Ke Za Zhi. 1995;33(7):406–8.
31. Huang YZ, Lu GZ, Zhao HS, et al. Clinical features and mortality-related factors of extensive burns among young adults: the Kunshan disaster experience. Ann Transl Med. 2020;8(17):1053. https://doi.org/10.21037/atm-20-288.
32. Shimizu R, Kishi K. Skin graft. Plast Surg Int. 2012;2012:563493. https://doi.org/10.1155/2012/563493.
33. Thompson JT, Marks MW. Negative pressure wound therapy. Clin Plast Surg. 2007;34(4):673–84. https://doi.org/10.1016/j.cps.2007.07.005.
34. Qiu X, Luo H, Huang G. Roles of negative pressure wound therapy for scar revision. Front Physiol. 2023;14:1194051. https://doi.org/10.3389/fphys.2023.1194051.
35. Rijpma D, Pijpe A, Claes K, et al. Outcomes of Meek micrografting versus mesh grafting on deep dermal and full thickness (burn) wounds: study protocol for an intra-patient randomized controlled trial. PLoS One. 2023;18(2):e0281347. https://doi.org/10.1371/journal.pone.0281347.
36. Pierpont YN, Dinh TP, Salas RE, et al. Obesity and surgical wound healing: a current review. Adv Wound Care. 2014;3(1):71–9. https://doi.org/10.1089/wound.2013.0473.
37. Frueh FS, Später T, Körbel C, et al. Prevascularization of dermal substitutes with adipose tissue-derived microvascular fragments enhances early skin grafting. Sci Rep. 2018;8:10977. https://doi.org/10.1038/s41598-018-29252-6.
38. Rapp SJ, Rumberg A, Visscher M, et al. Establishing a reproducible hypertrophic scar following thermal injury: a porcine model. Plast Reconstr Surg Glob Open. 2015;3(2):e309. https://doi.org/10.1097/GOX.0000000000000277.
39. Zhao JY, Chai JK, Song HF, Zhang J, Xu MH, Liang YD. Influence of hyaluronic acid on wound healing using composite porcine acellular dermal matrix grafts and autologous skin in rabbits. Int Wound J. 2013;5:562–72. https://doi.org/10.1111/j.1742-481X.2012.01023.x.
40. Raborn LN, Janis JE. Prevention and treatment of burn scar contracture: a practical review. Plast Reconstr Surg Glob Open. 2024;12(1):e5333. https://doi.org/10.1097/GOX.0000000000005333.
41. Ma Z, Mo R, Chen C, Meng X, Tan Q. Surgical treatment of joint burn scar contracture: a 10-year single-center experience with long-term outcome evaluation. Ann Transl Med. 2021;9(4):303. https://doi.org/10.21037/atm-20-4947.
42. Monstrey S, Middelkoop E, Vranckx JJ, Bassetto F, Ziegler UE, Meaume S, Téot L. Updated scar management practical guidelines: non-invasive and invasive measures. J Plast Reconstr Aesthet Surg. 2014;67(8):1017–25. https://doi.org/10.1016/j.bjps.2014.04.011.
43. Dogan S, Elmasry M, El-Serafi A, Sjöberg F, Vuola J, Kankuri E, Grigoriadi MP, Valtonen J, Abdelrahman I, Steinvall I, Karlsson M, Olofsson P, Lindford A. A prospective dual-centre intra-individual controlled study for the treatment of burns comparing dermis graft

with split-thickness skin auto-graft. Sci Rep. 2022;12(1):21666. https://doi.org/10.1038/s41598-022-25346-4.
44. Yammine K, Assi C. A meta-analysis of the outcomes of split-thickness skin graft on diabetic leg and foot ulcers. Int J Low Extrem Wounds. 2019;18(1):23–30. https://doi.org/10.1177/1534734619832123. Epub 2019 Mar 7
45. Vural E, Berbée M, Acott A, Blagg R, Fan CY, Hauer-Jensen M. Skin graft take rates, granulation, and epithelialization: dependence on myeloid cell hypoxia-inducible factor 1alpha. Arch Otolaryngol Head Neck Surg. 2010;136(7):720–3. https://doi.org/10.1001/archoto.2010.103.
46. Han TH, et al. The limited immunomodulatory effects of escharectomy on the kinetics of endotoxin, cytokines, and adhesion molecules in major burns. Mediat Inflamm. 2004;13(4):241–6.
47. McDougal WS, Slade CL, Pruitt BAJ. Manual of burns. New York: Springer-Verlag; 1978.
48. Herndon DN. Total burn care. Elsevier; 2017.
49. Yang Z. Burn therapeutics. Beijing: People's Medical Publishing House; 2006.
50. Bickell WH, et al. Immediate versus delayed fluid resuscitation for hypotensive patients with penetrating torso injuries. N Engl J Med. 1994;331(17):1105–9.
51. Williams-Johnson JA, et al. Effects of tranexamic acid on death, vascular occlusive events, and blood transfusion in trauma patients with significant haemorrhage (CRASH-2) a randomised, placebo-controlled trial. West Indian Med J. 2010;59(6):612–24.
52. Spahn DR, et al. Management of bleeding and coagulopathy following major trauma: an updated European guideline. Crit Care. 2013;17(2):R76.
53. Gelman S, Mushlin PS. Catecholamine-induced changes in the splanchnic circulation affecting systemic hemodynamics. Anesthesiology. 2004;100(2):434–9.
54. Guly HR, et al. Vital signs and estimated blood loss in patients with major trauma: testing the validity of the ATLS classification of hypovolaemic shock. Resuscitation. 2011;82(5):556–9.
55. Steadman PB, Pegg SP. A quantitative assessment of blood loss in burn wound excision and grafting. Burns. 1992;18(6):490–1.
56. Domínguez A, et al. Transfusion requirements in burn patients undergoing primary wound excision: effect of tranexamic acid. Minerva Anestesiol. 2017;83(4):353–60.
57. Atiyeh BS, Gunn SW, Hayek SN. State of the art in burn treatment. World J Surg. 2005;29(2):131–48.
58. Honari S. Topical therapies and antimicrobials in the management of burn wounds. Crit Care Nurs Clin North Am. 2004;16(1):1–11.
59. Church D, et al. Burn wound infections. Clin Microbiol Rev. 2006;19(2):403–34.
60. Moran KT, et al. A new algorithm for calculation of blood loss in excisional burn surgery. Am Surg. 1988;54(4):207–8.
61. Luo G, et al. Blood loss during extensive escharectomy and auto-microskin grafting in adult male major burn patients. Burns. 2011;37(5):790–3.
62. Budny PG, Regan PJ, Roberts AH. The estimation of blood loss during burns surgery. Burns. 1993;19(2):134–7.
63. Warden GD, Saffle JR, Kravitz M. A two-stage technique for excision and grafting of burn wounds. J Trauma. 1982;22(2):98–103.
64. Sihler KC, Napolitano LM. Complications of massive transfusion. Chest. 2010;137(1):209–20.
65. Sauaia A, et al. Early predictors of postinjury multiple organ failure. Arch Surg. 1994;129(1):39–45.
66. Palmieri TL. Burn injury and blood transfusion. Curr Opin Anaesthesiol. 2019;32(2):247–51.
67. Yamamoto T, Iwase H, King TW, et al. Skin xenotransplantation: historical review and clinical potential. Burns. 2018;44(7):1738–49. https://doi.org/10.1016/j.burns.2018.02.029.
68. Irilouzadian R, Khalaji A, Baghsheikhi H, et al. The clinical outcomes of xenografts in the treatment of burn patients: a systematic review and meta-analysis. Eur J Med Res. 2023;28(1):524. https://doi.org/10.1186/s40001-023-01505-9.
69. Chang LY, Yang JY, Chuang SS, et al. Use of the scalp as a donor site for large burn wound coverage: review of 150 patients. World J Surg. 1998;22(3):296–300. https://doi.org/10.1007/s002689900385.

70. Atiyeh BS, Costagliola M. Cultured epithelial autograft (CEA) in burn treatment: three decades later. Burns. 2007;33(4):405–13. https://doi.org/10.1016/j.burns.2006.11.002. Epub 2007 Apr 2
71. Medina A, Riegel T, Nystad D, et al. Modified Meek micrografting technique for wound coverage in extensive burn injuries. J Burn Care Res. 2016;37(5):305–13. https://doi.org/10.1097/BCR.0000000000000244.
72. Committee IPG, Steering S, Advisory S. Isbi practice guidelines for burn care. Burns. 2016;42(5):953–1021.
73. Liu Z, Li D, Liu X, et al. Elevated serum Procalcitonin to predict severity and prognosis of extensive burns. J Investig Surg. 2022;35(7):1510–8.
74. Resadita R, Seswandhana MR, Purnomo E, et al. The effect of Npwt in wound healing and bacterial count on deep dermal burn injury model: an experimental study. Ann Med Surg (Lond). 2022;75:103367.
75. Lin DZ, Kao YC, Chen C, et al. Negative pressure wound therapy for burn patients: a meta-analysis and systematic review. Int Wound J. 2021;18(1):112–23.
76. Nuhiji E. Trends and innovation in negative pressure wound therapy: a review of burn wound management. Adv Wound Care (New Rochelle). 2024;13(8):391–9.
77. Kantak NA, Mistry R, Varon DE, et al. Negative pressure wound therapy for burns. Clin Plast Surg. 2017;44(3):671–7.
78. Teng SC. Use of negative pressure wound therapy in burn patients. Int Wound J. 2016;13(Suppl 3):15–8.
79. Kantak NA, Mistry R, Halvorson EG. A review of negative-pressure wound therapy in the management of burn wounds. Burns. 2016;42(8):1623–33.
80. Ren Y, Chang P, Sheridan RL. Negative wound pressure therapy is safe and useful in pediatric burn patients. Int J Burns Trauma. 2017;7(2):12–6.
81. Kuromaru Y, Won P, Madrigal P, et al. Negative pressure wound therapy and its use in burn wounds: an updated systematic review. J Burn Care Res. 2025;46:581.
82. Zhaofan X. Multiple organ injury after burn and its prevention and treatment – one of the new advances in burn. Chinese J Burnss. 2006;22(3):164–7.
83. Zongcheng Y. Progress and prospect of severe burn treatment. Chinese J Burns. 2006;22(3):237–40.
84. Ding YL, et al. Clinical and histological observations on the application of intermingled auto- and porcine-skin heterografts in third degree burns. Burns Incl Therm Inj. 1983;9(6):381–6.
85. Lee SS, et al. "Shift to right flypaper technique" a refined method for postage stamp autografting preparation. Burns. 2007;33(6):764–9.
86. Shen ZA. Application of allogeneic skin in burn surgery. Zhonghua Shao Shang Za Zhi. 2019;35(4):243–7.
87. Jianhua C, et al. Establishment of fresh allogeneic scalp combined with autologous microparticle skin in the repair of limb wounds in patients with large-area burns and its curative effect. Chinese J Burns. 2019;35(4):253–60.
88. Zhang ML, et al. Microskin grafting in the treatment of extensive burns: a preliminary report. J Trauma. 1988;28(6):804–7.
89. Chen XL, et al. Microskin autografting in the treatment of burns over 70% of total body surface area: 14 years of clinical experience. Burns. 2011;37(6):973–80.
90. van der Veen VC, et al. Biological background of dermal substitutes. Burns. 2010;36(3):305–21.
91. Shen C, et al. Use of fresh scalp allografts from living relatives for extensive deep burns in children: a clinical study over 7 years. J Burn Care Res. 2021;42(2):323–30.
92. Chuanan S. Burn science: wound repair volume. Beijing: Science Press; 2020.
93. Cochrane T. The low temperature storage of skin: a preliminary report. Br J Plast Surg. 1968;21(2):118–25.
94. Baxter CR. Skin banking in the United States. J Burn Care Rehabil. 1985;6(4):322.
95. Blome-Eberwein S, et al. Clinical practice of glycerol preserved allograft skin coverage. Burns. 2002;28(Suppl 1):S10–2.

96. Ben-Bassat H. Performance and safety of skin allografts. Clin Dermatol. 2005;23(4):365–75.
97. Cai JH, et al. Effects of scar excision combined with negative-pressure on repair of hypertrophic scar in burn children. Zhonghua Shao Shang Za Zhi. 2017;33(7):410–4.
98. Collaboration, MEEK Micro-skin Transplantation Technology, and Chinese Burn Association Group. Clinical operation procedure of grafting technique of MEEK micro-skin. Zhonghua Shao Shang Za Zhi. 2019;35(8):561–4.
99. Zongcheng Y, Shiliang W. Li Ao burn therapeutics, version 3. Beijing: People's Medical Publishing House; 2006.

Chapter 4
New Methods for Prevention and Treatment of Complications

Chuanan Shen, Tianjun Sun, Bohan Zhang, Dongjie Li, Jianhua Cai, and Dawei Li

4.1 Infections Associated with Catheters and Tubes

4.1.1 Improving the Management of Catheters and Tubes

[Background]

Though the incidence of burn wound sepsis has decreased with the continuous progress of dressing techniques, medications, and dressing materials, infections and even sepsis associated with catheters and tubes have become more prevalent with the precise management in intensive care medicine [1]. Annually, approximately 80,000 patients in United States intensive care units experience catheter-related infections, with a resulting mortality rate of approximately 12–25% [2]. Patients with extensive burn injuries, characterized by compromised immune systems, are particularly susceptible to infections. In burn intensive care units in China, the infection rate stands at as high as 30 per 1000 catheter-days, with catheter-related sepsis emerging as a primary cause of mortality among patients with extensive burns [3].

In response to this challenge, we have implemented a set of guidelines for catheter and tube use to effectively mitigate the risk of catheter- and tube-related sepsis.

Technical Points
Central Venous Catheters

Central venous catheters may be inserted either centrally or peripherally, depending on the clinical context. The guiding principles in our practice include:

C. Shen (✉) · T. Sun · B. Zhang · D. Li · J. Cai · D. Li
The Medical Department of Burn and Plastic Surgery, The 4th Medical Center, PLAGH, Beijing, China

C. Shen (ed.), *Novel Strategies for Critical Burn Care*,
https://doi.org/10.1007/978-981-92-0325-3_4

- Central venous catheterization is generally avoided during fluid resuscitation in the burn shock stage if peripheral venous access is feasible.
- A central line is required during major eschar excision procedures to facilitate the infusion of large fluid volumes and to prepare for potential emergent interventions. However, careful consideration is essential to determine the postoperative necessity of retaining the catheter.
- Peripheral veins are the preferred initial choice for venous access in routine care. Should central venous access be required, a peripherally inserted central catheter (PICC) is favored due to its lower infection risk.
- Utilizing total enteral nutrition can help reduce the reliance on central venous catheter use.

Arterial Catheter

- Arterial catheterization is typically avoided during fluid resuscitation in the burn shock stage.
- An arterial catheter is inserted during major surgical procedures and is to be removed once the patient has emerged from anesthesia and demonstrates stable blood pressure.
- An indwelling arterial line is reserved for critical patients with fluctuating blood pressure. However, it should be promptly removed upon stabilization of the patient's condition.

Tracheotomy Tube

- Removal of a tracheotomy tube is recommended once the airway edema subsides.
- Fiberoptic bronchoscopy can be utilized to monitor airway mucosal swelling and shedding, assessing the risk of airway obstruction to inform extubation decisions.
- Assessment of lung function and overall patient status guides the determination of the necessity for prolonged mechanical ventilation and subsequent extubation considerations.
- Prolonged retention of a tracheotomy tube solely for anesthetic convenience is discouraged.

Urinary Catheter

- A urinary catheter should be placed to monitor the hourly urine output in patient undergoing resuscitation, but as soon as the patient has emerged from the burn shock stage and the hourly urine output no longer needs to be monitored for the adequacy of resuscitation, the catheter should be removed, unless dysuria is a concern.
- Subsequent catheterization may be warranted for specific interventions like surgery, but extended catheter retention is discouraged for prolonged periods.

Nasogastric Tube

A nasogastric tube is indicated for gastrointestinal decompression or feeding in the initial stages following a burn injury. However, ongoing assessment is essential as the patient's nutritional requirements diminish with the reduction in wound size.

Ideally, oral intake should be prioritized over nasogastric tube feeding whenever feasible.

[Typical Case]

The patient, a 3-year-old girl, sustained multiple flame burns during a gas leakage and explosion accident. She was immediately sent to a local hospital where she received fluid resuscitation through left femoral vein catheterization and wound cleaning. Subsequently, she was transferred to our center where she underwent tracheotomy and escharotomy in the ED 14 h post-injury.

Specialized Physical Examination: The patient presents with burn injuries covering approximately 85% TBSA, with sparing of skin noted in specific areas such as the anterior trunk (adjacent to the neck, umbilical region, and thighs), posterior trunk, and axillae. The majority of wounds exhibit a pale and leathery appearance, while those on the face, neck, and lower extremities appear red and white with excessive exudate. Her mouth resembled the semirigid mouth of the fish. The tracheotomy tube was well fixed, unobstructed, and connected to a respiratory filter. The left femoral vein catheter was in place and unobstructed.

Admission Diagnoses: ① Burn injuries: 85% TBSA, comprising 30% TBSA second-degree burns and 55% TBSA third-degree burns, ② Inhalation injury, ③ Post-tracheotomy status, ④ Water-electrolyte imbalance, ⑤ Coagulation abnormalities, and ⑥ Hypoproteinemia.

The management of the patient's catheters, i.e., the central venous catheter, the arterial catheter, the tracheotomy tube, the urinary catheter, and the nasogastric tube, adhered to established protocols. Notably, the patient did not experience any catheter- and tube-related infections or sepsis. The treatment course proceeded smoothly and resulted in a successful outcome. Details regarding the catheter applications are illustrated in Fig. 4.1.

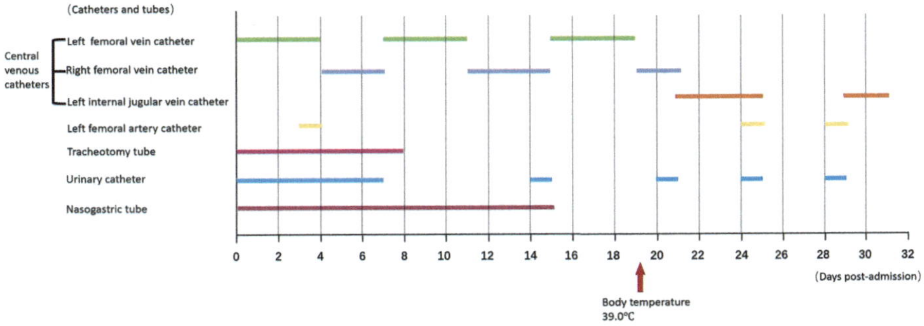

Fig. 4.1 Patient catheter management

[Discussion]

In the management of large burns, the decision to retain catheters or tubes must be meticulously assessed based on individual circumstances. It is of great significance to reduce the incidence of catheter- or tube-related infection. Different catheters and tubes may lead to different risks in different patients. Central venous and arterial catheterization through burn wounds would increase the risk of infection, necessitating careful selection of catheterization sites and timely site rotation [4]. Furthermore, vigilance is essential to prevent tracheotomy tube-related infections and potential complications like tracheoesophageal fistula or tracheal stenosis from factors such as granulation tissue formation. Regular monitoring and assessment are imperative [5, 6]. Prolonged use of urinary catheters in female patients can predispose them to urinary tract infections, underscoring the importance of minimizing unnecessary catheterization duration [7, 8]. Strategies such as catheter clamping and bladder training prior to catheter removal may be implemented to mitigate the risk of re-catheterization [9].

Over the past years, our team has adhered to these guidelines in managing diverse catheters and tubes for patients with extensive burns. Specifically, we have limited the duration of indwelling central venous catheters to a maximum of 3 days consecutively, with a total duration not exceeding 11 days; arterial catheters are retained for no longer than 1 day consecutively and up to 3 days cumulatively; mechanical ventilation through tracheostomy tubes is restricted to 8 days; indwelling urinary catheters, 9 days consecutively, and within 23 days totally. These measures have significantly reduced both catheter durations and associated infections.

(Chuanan Shen, Tianjun Sun, Bohan Zhang)

4.1.2 Arterial Catheter

[Background]

Invasive arterial blood pressure monitoring using an arterial catheter provides real-time and accurate assessments of blood pressure levels [10]. It is utilized in major surgery, critical patients with unstable hemodynamics, cardiopulmonary resuscitation, and other special conditions [11–13]. Common catheterization sites include the dorsalis pedis artery, ulnar and radial arteries, brachial artery, and femoral artery. In patients with extensive burns, where the four extremities are often affected and may require surgical intervention, the groin area is frequently chosen for femoral artery catheterization [14]. The femoral artery, being a major vessel with an approximate inner diameter of 8 mm, is readily accessible for catheterization [15]. Currently, the standard arterial catheter used is a 20G needle (1.10 mm × 45 mm). However, when establishing a femoral artery line, patient edema can limit the length of the catheter within the vessel, increasing the risks of kinking, occlusion, dislodgement, etc. [16].

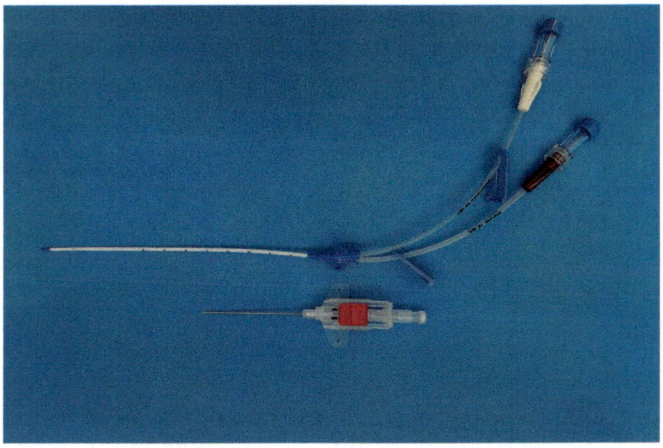

Fig. 4.2 Comparison of 5F pediatric central venous catheter and 20G arterial indwelling needle

In recent years, our team has explored the use of a pediatric central venous catheter (5F × 13 cm, with inner diameters of 20G and 18G for the two lumens, respectively) for femoral artery catheterization. Our findings indicate that this approach has provided stable and reliable performance in intraoperative blood pressure monitoring (see Fig. 4.2).

[Protocol]
Patient Assessment

The patient's vital signs, level of consciousness, burn wound conditions, availability of peripheral arteries, and conditions of the potential femoral artery puncture site are comprehensively assessed. The femoral artery line is considered only after all alternatives have been ruled out.

Technical Points

- Strictly follow the principles of sterile technique: perform hand hygiene, and wear disposable surgical gown, masks, caps, and gloves.
- Apply iodophor antiseptic to the skin surrounding the puncture site in a circular motion, starting from the center and moving outward to a radius of 15–20 cm, followed by placing a sterile fenestrated drape.
- Avoid repeated attempts at catheterization; utilize ultrasound guidance for puncture if necessary.
- A sharp blade can be used to carefully incise the eschar if the puncture site is covered with tough eschar. Insert the catheter gently and swiftly. Avoid violent injuries to the site.
- Position the patient supine, ensuring the hips are elevated to fully expose and tauten the skin in the groin area.
- Insertion of the spring-wire guide should only commence once successful access to the femoral artery with the introducer needle is confirmed. Remove the spring-wire guide assembly promptly after catheter insertion.

- Immediately clamp the catheter following successful insertion, and perform a pulsatile flush with heparinized saline to maintain patency.
- Secure the catheter wings to the burn wound with sutures.
- Dress the insertion site with iodine-impregnated gauze. A film dressing can be applied if normal skin is available in the surrounding area.
- Minimize the duration of catheter use; remove it as soon as blood pressure stabilizes.
- After extubation, press the insertion site for 10 ~ 15 min, and use sandbags for continued compression if indicated.

[Typical Case]

Patient Profile: A 20-year-old male sustained extensive flame burns resulting from gas leakage and explosion, presenting at our center approximately 3 h post-injury.

Admission Diagnoses: ① Burn size, 80%TBSA; burn depth, degree II ~ III, and ② inhalation injury.

Treatment Protocol: Upon admission, the patient received immediate fluid resuscitation, escharotomy, intensive care management, and comprehensive nutritional support.

Surgical Intervention: Three major operations were performed to repair the deep burn wounds on both upper extremities, both lower extremities and trunks.

Catheterization Management: A pediatric central venous catheter was utilized for femoral artery catheterization during surgical interventions. The catheter was removed within 2 h postoperatively. No subsequent complications such as dislodgement, tube occlusion, tube crimping, infection, or femoral artery bleeding were observed.

[Discussion]

Femoral artery catheterization for invasive arterial blood pressure monitoring is often preferred for operations for extensive burn patients [17]. The complex nature of these procedures, characterized by large eschar excision, significant blood loss, and substantial fluid requirements, necessitates precise hemodynamic monitoring [18, 19]. We reviewed 118 adult cases of extensive burns that received artery catheterization with pediatric 5F double lumen central venous catheter in our center and found that this approach demonstrated exceptional procedural safety, with no instances of crimping, occlusion, dislodgement or complications such as postoperative bleeding and catheter-related infections.

The advantages of using pediatric 5F central venous catheter for arterial monitoring include: ① Procedural Efficacy. High catheterization success rate. Steps of this procedure are similar to that of femoral vein catheterization. ② Catheter Characteristics. Polyurethane material facilitates smooth vessel advancement, minimal thrombus formation, reduced vessel wall irritation and provides ease of radiographic positioning confirmation. ③ Technical Specifications. A length of 13cm makes it easy to suture the catheter in place to avoid dislodgment, particularly for patients with obesity or edema. ④ Functional Benefits. Double-lumen design supporting comprehensive blood gas analysis.

However, it also has limitations such as higher cost, risks of increased bleeding during insertion and extubation [20]. Often, experienced physician intervention is required, sterile techniques are strictly adhered, timely removal preferred, and complications carefully monitored.

(Chuanan Shen, Dongjie Li)

4.2 Gastrointestinal Hemorrhage

4.2.1 Application of NPWT to Prevent Infections and Promote Healing of Both Surgical Incision and Burn Wounds in Patients with Massive GI Bleeding

[Background]
Stress ulcer can induce acute erosions and ulcers in esophagus and gastrointestinal tract. In critical cases, it may precipitate gastrointestinal bleeding, perforation, and acute peritonitis, thus exacerbating the clinical scenario substantially. Stress ulcers that occur 1~3 weeks post-major burns are also known as Curling's ulcers [21]. Although the reported incidence rates are variable [22–24], a steady increase in detection rates has been observed, courtesy of advancements in fiberoptic gastroscopy, and other diagnostic methodologies. That said, massive hemorrhage in conjunction with perforation is uncommon in burn patients, and the development of a duodenal perforation into the retroperitoneum is a rare event. Once it occurs, the perforation site exhibits an elevated risk of fistula formation, potentially leading to intra-abdominal infections. Concurrently, the insertion of multiple abdominal drainage tubes escalates the risk of infection from these openings and the mortality rate. This clinical scenario is further complicated in the presence of extensive deep abdominal burn injuries. Curling's ulcers predominantly manifest in the early stage postburn, and the earlier their onset, the more profound the impact on the patient's overall condition. A substantial volume of blood loss and subsequent blood transfusion can precipitate a series of severe complications such as ischemia-reperfusion injury and coagulation dysfunction. This denies many deep burn wounds the opportunity to receive timely and effective coverage. Furthermore, deep abdominal burns escalate the risk of both intra-abdominal infections and the infection of surgical incision made to address ulcers or hemorrhaging. The situation is further exacerbated as, during these stages, patient nutrition is primarily dependent on parenteral administration via venous catheters, thereby significantly increasing the risk of catheter-related sepsis.

In the management of these patients, we have employed negative pressure wound treatment (NPWT) [25] to prevent potential adverse outcomes such as incision dehiscence and omental tissue exposure, reduce the risk of drainage tube-associated infections, and promote the healing of both deep burn wounds and surgical incisions. The method has demonstrated efficacy and satisfactory performance in our clinical practice.

Key Technical Points

- The abdominal surgery incision and the surrounding wound together should be covered with the NPWT material after careful debridement. To achieve a firm coverage, the method of tension reduction and fixation is often used (see Sect. 3.3.2 of Chap. 3: Phased Excision and Suture of Deep Burn Wound).
- The entrance site of the drainage tubes should be completely sealed with NPWT material. However, it should be noted that the material would contract when negative pressure is applied. Therefore, sufficient room should be made for the tubes to avoid compression which could impede drainage.
- In cases without enough unaffected skin for the NPWT film to attach, commercially available xenografts can be applied to the neighboring eschar tissue and dried with a dryer to promote adherence, and then the film can be stapled to the dried xenografts to create a satisfactory negative pressure environment. If the wound that is to be applied with NPWT happens to neighbor burned perineum, the perineum area can also be sealed in after placement of a urinary catheter (Fig. 4.3). Careful attention should be paid to potential negative pressure leakage caused by the maceration of edge tissues. Negative pressure leakage needs immediate response.

The patient had no unaffected skin in the thighs, and xenografts were used for NPWT materials to attach. The xenografts were placed at the root of the thighs and dried to adhere tightly. Then NPWT films were applied to the xenografts to form a sealed environment. The patient's perineum with burn injury was also sealed in after placement of a urinary catheter.

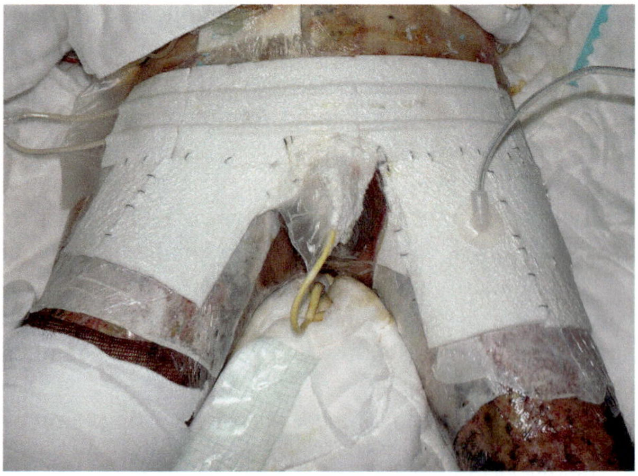

Fig. 4.3 Placement of NPWT with the assistance of xenografts

- NPWT drainage tube is easy to be blocked by blood clots in the early stage after operation. It should be cleared frequently and replaced when necessary.
- Timely renewal of the NPWT dressings should be performed. For obviously contaminated wounds, the dressings are generally renewed within 2–3 days and for cleaner wounds 5–7 days.
- Flushing of the NPWT dressings should be avoided to prevent intra-abdominal infections.
- A continuous and aggressive intra-abdominal flushing and drainage can minimize the risk of intra-abdominal infection. It is imperative to ensure that the drainage tube is unobstructed. It should be noted that even during surgeries for burn wounds, a continuous intra-abdominal drainage under negative pressure is essential.
- The flushing fluid should be heated to 37 °C to prevent stimulation from a large amount of cold fluid. Flushing should be done in a rapid and continuous pattern to avoid blockage of the drainage tubes as much as possible.

Other Treatments

After the surgery, the patient can be gradually given glucose and sodium chloride solution, rice soup, enteral nutrition emulsions, etc., through nasogastric tube feeding after normal flatulence. If the surgical incision heals smoothly, the patient can return to a normal diet. On the contrary, if a fistula forms, the patient's vital signs, localized symptoms, laboratory, and other test results should be carefully monitored, and conservative treatment with NPWT and continuous abdominal irrigation or another emergency laparotomy may be needed. During the conservative treatment, all nutrition is given parenterally, the total amount of intravenous infusion should be carefully assessed to avoid inflicting excessive cardiopulmonary load, various vitamins and trace elements in addition to glucose, amino acids, and fat emulsion should be administrated, and the care for the central venous line should be strengthened to minimize the risk of catheter-related sepsis.

[Typical Case]

The patient, a 50-year-old man who suffered extensive burns due to contact with high voltage electricity (10,000 V), was sent to a local hospital 3 h after the injury where he was diagnosed with deep second-degree to third-degree burns with a total burn size of 70% TBSA. He received anti-shock and anti-infection treatment, organ protection, nutritional support, debridement, and surgical treatment for part of the wounds. Gastrointestinal bleeding was first observed on the tenth post-injury day in the form of hematochezia with a blood loss volume of about 1000 mL. In the following week, intermittent hematemesis and hematochezia occurred with a maximum blood loss of 4000 mL. He was transferred to our center on the 16th day after the injury.

Upon admission, the patient was emaciated, anemic, and febrile with a body temperature of 38.6 °C. Auscultation found obvious moist rales in both lungs and active bowel sounds in the abdomen. The burn size was about 70% TBSA. Some wounds on the top of the head, abdomen, and buttocks were covered with yellowish white necrotic tissue, and the rest of the wounds were covered with dark and partly charred eschar. Allogeneic skin grafts could be seen on both lower extremities. Some of the grafts took well, and some had macerated with purulent secretions under them. Grafts on the legs were in poorer condition, with grafts in the right leg dried and dead, closely adhering to the tibia (Fig. 4.4a). Lab tests showed: white blood cell count, 15.01×10^9/L; neutrophil percentage, 91.4%; red blood cell count, 3.65×10^{12}/L; hemoglobin, 112 g/L; platelet count, 151×10^9/L; blood potassium, 3.23 mmol/L; blood sodium, 153 mmol/L; blood chlorine, 112 mmol/L; procalcitonin, 18.88 ng/mL; and brain natriuretic peptide, 1896 pg/mL. Chest X-ray and CT suggested bilateral lung infection, atelectasis with pleural effusion, and pelvic effusion. The patient denied ulcer or other underlying diseases.

Admission Diagnosis: ① burn size, 70% TBSA; burn depth, deep II degree (20%TBSA), III degree (44%TBSA) and IV degree (6%TBSA), ② Gastrointestinal bleeding, ③ pulmonary infection, ④ bilateral atelectasis, ⑤ bilateral pleural effusion, ⑥ peritoneal effusion, ⑦ pelvic effusion, and ⑧ electrolyte imbalance

Treatment Course: The patient was instructed to stop food and drinks. Continuous infusion of somatostatin and esomeprazole, supplements of blood products, and parenteral nutritional products were given. The patient had episodes of hematemesis and hematochezia in the evening on the admission day, with a blood loss volume of about 1600 mL. These symptoms were relieved with treatment, but after that melena still occurred every day subsequently. On the evening of the 25th day postburn, the patient had a severe episode of hematochezia and hematemesis, resulting in a blood loss of about 1200 mL and shock, which did not respond well to conservative treatment. Bedside gastroscopy revealed a huge duodenal hematoma with active bleeding (Fig. 4.4b). After multidisciplinary consultation and discussion with gastroenterologists, general surgeon, and interventionists, emergency exploratory laparotomy was performed in the early morning of the next day. The laparotomy found a 3 cm × 3 cm rupture at the proximal end of the horizontal part of the duodenum and the resultant huge retroperitoneal hematoma with a volume of about 3000 mL and pus coating inside the cavity wall. Billroth's II operation, sew-up of the rupture, and ostomy surgery were performed. Subphrenic drainage tubes were placed. The duodenal cut end, the lowest point of retroperitoneal cavity, and left side of the pelvic floor also received drainage tubes. An NG tube, an NJ tube, a duodenostomy tube, and a cholecystostomy tube were also placed (Fig. 4.4c). The abdominal incision, stoma, and the neighboring abdominal wounds were sealed with NPWT materials (Fig. 4.4d) with drainage tubes connected to the central negative pressure system that provides negative pressure between −59.8 and −79.8kpa. The abdominal cavity was continuously irrigated with copious normal saline, furacilin solutions, and gentamicin-saline solution. After flatulence, the patient was gradually given glucose and sodium chloride solution, rice soup, and nutrition emulsion through the tube feeding. Subsequently, the tubes except the one for

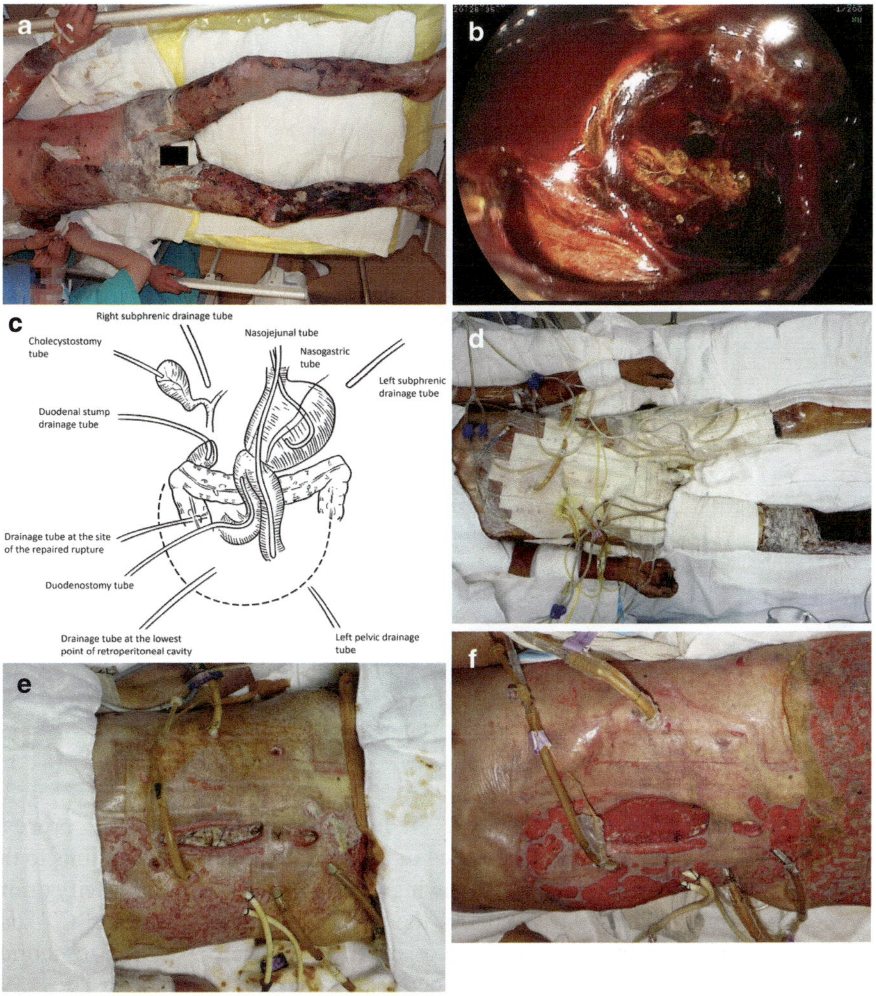

Fig. 4.4 Treatment of a patient who sustained high-voltage electrical burns and developed retroperitoneal perforation and severe gastrointestinal bleeding. (**a**) The overall wound condition upon admission. (**b**) Gastroscopy showed huge duodenal hematoma with active bleeding. (**c**) Schematic diagram of drainage tube placement after laparotomy. (**d**) The surgical incision, stomas, and excised wounds were dressed with NPWT materials. (**e**) The abdominal incision partly dehisced. (**f**) With negative pressure treatment, the necrotic tissue of incision dehiscence was eventually removed, and fresh granulation tissue could be seen (a photo taken on the 56th day post-injury). (**g**) The incision eventually healed after grafting. (**h**) 31 days after the exploratory laparotomy, the wounds were clean under negative pressure treatment and the grafts survived. (**i**) Patient in good recovery

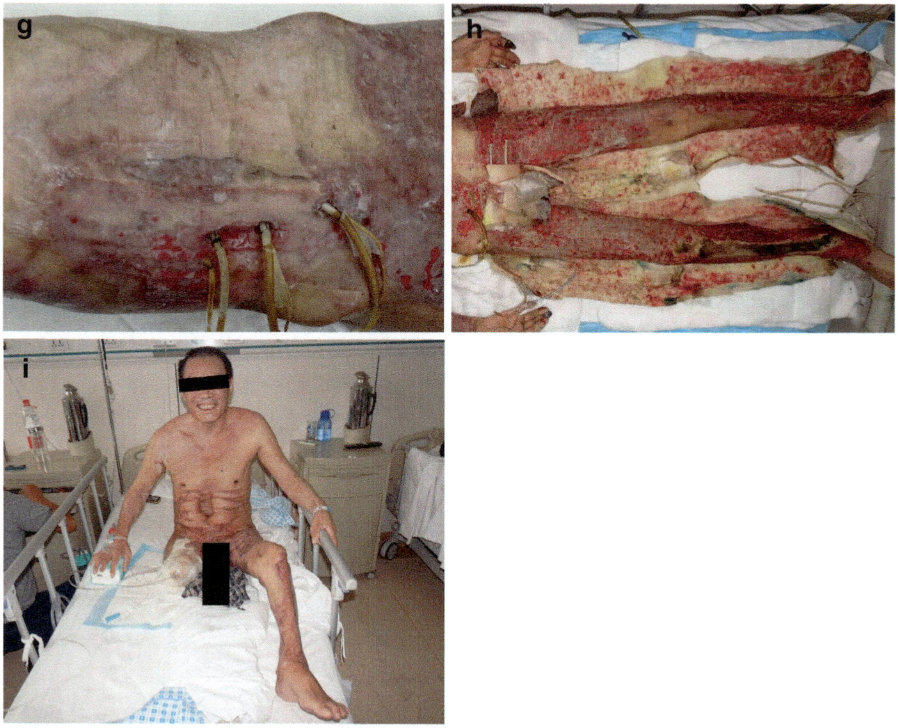

Fig. 4.4 (continued)

retroperitoneal cavity drainage were gradually removed. During the process, despite all efforts to identify the source of the symptom and modifications to the therapy, chyme-like contents kept showing up in the retroperitoneal cavity drainage tube. On the 127th day postburn, the patient developed fever and CT scan suggested effusion in the right iliac fossa. An emergency operation to debride and drain the abdominal abscess was performed.

During the operation, about 150 mL thin pus was found within the right retroperitoneal cavity, not affecting the abdominal cavity. To deal with this, two dual-lumen drainage tubes were placed at the lowest point of the sump. After closure, all drainage tubes, surgical incision, and the residual burn wounds were dressed with NPWT materials, and continuous irrigation and drainage were carried out. The particular drainage and wound conditions were carefully inspected, and the NPWT materials were regularly changed. During the process, the patient's surgical incision in the median section partly dehisced, exposing the internal omental tissue

(Fig. 4.4e). Fortunately, with continuous negative pressure treatment, granulation tissue gradually forms around the dehiscence (Fig. 4.4f) and provided good conditions for skin grafting (Fig. 4.4g). All wounds healed eventually and no serious abdominal infection or other adverse complications occurred during the treatment.

Due to extensive exposure of the right tibia, the right knee, and the right ankle which were also complicated with suppurative arthritis, the patient received above-the-knee amputation for the right lower limb. All the wounds were treated with intermingled transplantation of auto- and allografts, sealed with NPWT materials to facilitate drainage and promote healing (Fig. 4.4h). The wounds gradually healed, part of the abdominal drainage tubes were removed, and the patient was transferred to the Department of General Surgery on the 158th day postburn. Eventually, all the abdominal drainage tubes were gradually removed, and the patient was discharged (Fig. 4.4i).

[Discussion]

Gastrointestinal bleeding is a common complication of large burns [22–24]. For most cases, such bleeding can be controlled with conservative treatment, but in cases of arterial bleeding or intestinal perforation, laparotomy is necessary and inevitably will complicate the situation, particularly when the abdomen is also burnt since this puts the drainage site at a higher risk of infection and makes the incision less likely to heal. NPWT provides a closed space with negative pressure which promotes efficient unidirectional drainage and lowers the risks of abdominal cavity infection caused by pollution through the drainage openings and the surgical incision from the surrounding burn wounds and the external environment [25]. Additionally, NPWT also helps to reduce the tension around the abdominal incision to lower the risk of incision dehiscence.

For cases with difficulties to deploy negative pressure materials on wound surface, allografts, exhibiting property of tight adherence to wound surface after drying, can be used as "cushions" to which the NPWT materials can be applied.

As for the burn wounds, repeated debridement plus regular renewal of NPWT materials speed the removal of necrotic tissue and provide effective coverage for the wounds, minimizing infection for the patient. Additionally, the NPWT dressings with full contact with the wounds can drain the exudates as much as possible, reducing local swelling and eliminating inflammatory mediators, lactic acid and other substances with the exudate, so as to promote wound healing.

Therefore, with the proper application of NPWT, the risk of dehiscence of the abdominal surgical incision is minimized, the survival of the skin grafts for burn treatment is enhanced and the overall patient recovery is promoted.

(Chuanan Shen, Jianhua Cai)

4.3 The Use of Blood Products

[Background]

Anemia, hypoalbuminemia, and hypoglobulinemia are frequent complications of large burns [26]. Anemia undermines the oxygen-carrying capacity of the blood, leading to systemic oxygen deficiency. This, in turn, results in reduced energy levels, diminished appetite, and delayed wound healing. Hypoalbuminemia, characterized by an abnormally low level of albumin in the blood, reduces the colloid osmotic pressure, contributing to generalized tissue edema. This edema not only impedes wound healing but also disrupts normal organ function [27]. Similarly, hypoglobulinemia weakens the immune system, rendering the patient more susceptible to infections [28, 29]. Given the significant impact of these conditions on burn recovery, timely and effective correction of anemia, hypoalbuminemia, and hypoglobulinemia—typically through blood transfusions—is critical in the management of large burns [30]. However, in clinical practice, treatment protocols for these complications can vary, and they are sometimes insufficiently emphasized.

In our work, we place a strong emphasis on the prevention and treatment of anemia, hypoalbuminemia, and hypoglobulinemia, recognizing their pivotal roles in improving patient outcomes and promoting recovery.

[Protocol]

Close monitoring of hemoglobin, albumin, and globulin levels in the patient's blood is essential, with appropriate supplementation to maintain these parameters within their physiological range.

Blood transfusion. The infusion of red blood cell suspension remains the most direct and effective method for correcting anemia. Minimizing blood loss during surgical procedures, dressing changes, and preventing gastrointestinal bleeding are all important measures to reduce the incidence of anemia. It is generally recommended to maintain hemoglobin levels at a physiological range, with a target of no less than 110 g/L.

Supplementation of albumin and globulin. Albumin and globulin levels should be maintained at no less than 35 g/L and 30 g/L, respectively, to ensure proper oncotic pressure and substance transportation and immune function.

Whole blood transfusion. Transfusion should provide what has been lost. Patients with large burns often experience a large amount of whole blood loss during major surgery; therefore, fresh whole blood transfusion is advised. The benefits of fresh whole blood transfusion are particularly pronounced in patients with severe infections and significant metabolic depletion.

[Typical Case]

The patient, a 67-year-old man, presented to our center 1 h following multiple flame burns sustained in a natural gas explosion.

Admission Diagnoses: ① burn size, 90% TBSA; burn depths, third degree (75%), deep second degree (12%) and shallow second degree (3%), ② emphysema, and ③ hypoalbuminemia.

Specialized Physical Examination: The patient presented burn wounds with a total size of 90% TBSA (Fig. 4.5). Unaffected skin (10%TBSA) was seen in the occipital region, the right upper and lower extremity, the right lateral back, the buttock, and the perineum. Mild hoarseness, scorched hair, eyebrows and nasal hairs, and a small amount of black particles can be seen in the nasal cavity and sputum. He reported no tenderness upon palpation of most wound areas. Wounds on the face, neck, and lower extremities appeared red and white with significant exudation. The patient exhibited cold extremities, severe eyelid, and conjunctival swelling.

Treatment: Upon admission, the patient was provided with intensive burn care, including fluid resuscitation, infection control, organ function protection, total enteral nutritional support, and immune support. He underwent wound debridement and dressing changes, received transfusions of appropriate blood products (as detailed in Table 4.1), and had surgeries as scheduled. In particular, transfusions of whole blood, RBC suspension, albumin, and gamma globulin were performed, and for most of the patient's stay, his hemoglobin, albumin, and globulin levels were maintained at no less than 110 g/L, 35 g/L, and 30 g. The patient eventually recovered (Fig. 4.6).

(Chuanan Shen)

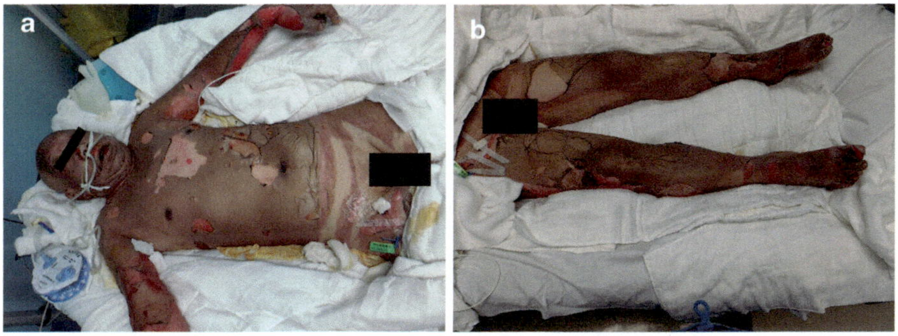

Fig. 4.5 (**a**) Wounds of the anterior trunk upon admission. (**b**) Wound of the lower extremities upon admission

Table 4.1 Use of blood products for the patient

		Transfusion of whole blood products				Lab test results			
Day post-injury	Whole blood (mL)	Red blood cell (U)	Plasma (mL)	Albumin (g)	Gamma globulin (g)	Hemoglobin (g/L)	Albumin (g/L)	Globulin (g/L)	Operation day
1st	/	/	2120	20	/	140	24.4	24.7	
2nd	/	/	2620	20	/	143	30.2	21.1	
3rd	1200	2	2000	20	/	108	32.3	25.9	Yes
4th	/	4	600	10	20	97	31.6	25.3	
5th	2000	/	1600	10	25	111	31.4	31.3	Yes
6th	800	/	750	20	20	108	33.1	25.5	
7th	/	/	1100	40	/	121	34.8	31.5	
8th	/	/	1400	20	/	119	34	28.4	
9th	400	/	1000	20	/	114	36.9	28.1	
10th	200	/	500	40	10	120	36.1	26.6	
11th	400	/	400	40	5	111	36.1	27.8	
12th	400	/	800	60	10	117	36.2	28.1	
13th	200	/	600	40	10	115	39.4	26.1	
14th	400	/	600	40	5	111	35.4	30.1	
15th	400	/	600	40	5	115	37.1	30.3	
16th	/	/	400	20	5	118	34.5	30.5	
17th	200	/	600	40	/	115	36.3	31.1	
18th	/	/	600	40	/	118	37.2	31.4	

19th	/	/	600	40	5	115	34.4	28.6	
20th	/	/	600	40	5	114	35.3	29.1	
21st	540	/	400	40	/	108	34.1	28.4	
22nd	/	/	800	40	10	113	34.6	32.9	
23rd	/	/	800	40	5	118	34.4	33.3	
24th	1600	/	2800	40	5	107	33.8	28.4	Yes
25th	400	/	1000	20	5	99	35.2	26.8	
26th	/	4	800	20	10	103	34.2	30.4	

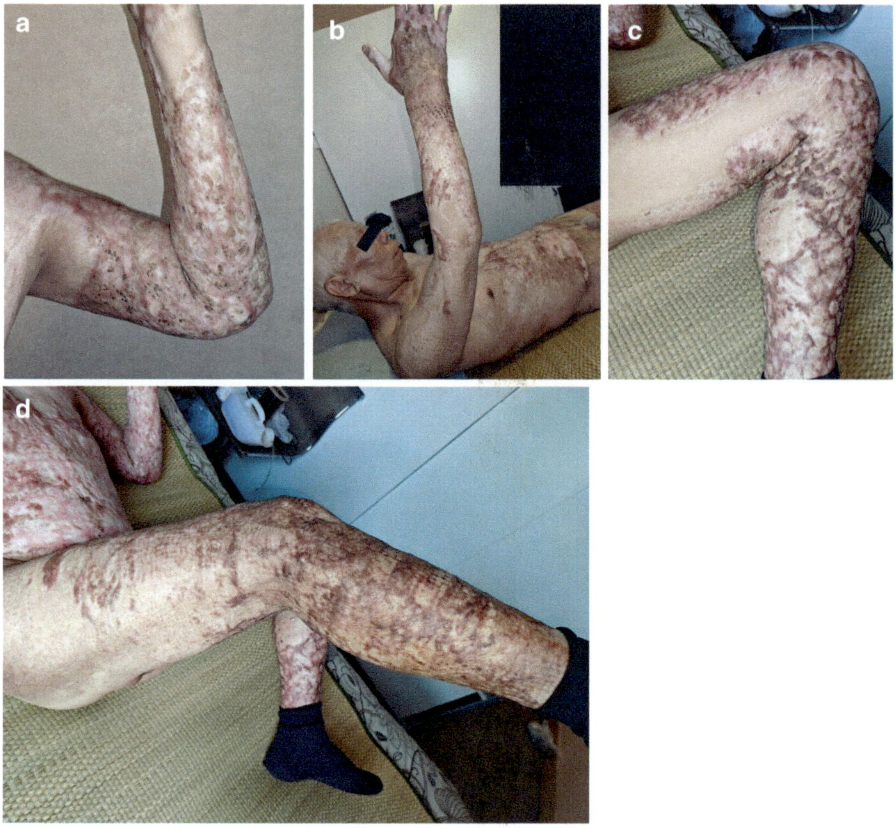

Fig. 4.6 (**a**) Satisfactory functional restoration of the left upper extremity (10 months post-surgery). (**b**) Satisfactory functional restoration of the right upper extremity (10 months post-surgery). (**c**) Satisfactory functional restoration of the left lower extremity (10 months post-surgery). (**d**) Satisfactory functional restoration of the right lower extremity (10 months post-surgery)

References

1. Hranjec T, Sawyer RG. Management of infections in critically ill patients. Surg Infect. 2014;15(5):474–8.
2. Heybati K, et al. Catheter management across patients with hematologic malignancies and catheter-related blood stream infections: a systematic review. Ann Hematol. 2022;101(11):2515–24.
3. Luo XQ, et al. Analysis of distribution and drug resistance of pathogens isolated from 159 patients with catheter-related bloodstream infection in burn intensive care unit. Zhonghua Shao Shang Za Zhi. 2020;36(1):24–31.
4. Buetti N, Timsit JF. Management and prevention of central venous catheter-related infections in the ICU. Semin Respir Crit Care Med. 2019;40(4):508–23.
5. Chua AP, Dalal B, Mehta AC. Tracheostomy tube-induced tracheoesophageal fistula. J Bronchol Interv Pulmonol. 2009;16(3):191–2.
6. Lal DR, Oldham KT. Recurrent tracheoesophageal fistula. Eur J Pediatr Surg. 2013;23(3):214–8.

7. Chen YY, et al. Using a criteria-based reminder to reduce use of indwelling urinary catheters and decrease urinary tract infections. Am J Crit Care. 2013;22(2):105–14.
8. Janzen J, et al. Reduction of unnecessary use of indwelling urinary catheters. BMJ Qual Saf. 2013;22(12):984–8.
9. Millner R, Becknell B. Urinary tract infections. Pediatr Clin N Am. 2019;66(1):1–13.
10. Saugel B, et al. How to measure blood pressure using an arterial catheter: a systematic 5-step approach. Crit Care. 2020;24(1):172.
11. Larsen EN, et al. A pilot randomised controlled trial of dressing and securement methods to prevent arterial catheter failure in intensive care. Aust Crit Care. 2021;34(1):38–46.
12. Yates AR, et al. Survival and cardiopulmonary resuscitation hemodynamics following cardiac arrest in children with surgical compared to medical heart disease. Pediatr Crit Care Med. 2019;20(12):1126–36.
13. Fieghen HE, et al. The hemodynamic tolerability and feasibility of sustained low efficiency dialysis in the management of critically ill patients with acute kidney injury. BMC Nephrol. 2010;11:32.
14. Tong Z, et al. An analysis of complications of brachial and axillary artery punctures. Am Surg. 2016;82(12):1250–6.
15. Turi ZG. Ending "poke until you get a gusher": Part II—the evidence based approach to vascular access revisited. Catheter Cardiovasc Interv. 2017;89(7):1193–4.
16. Paraggio L, et al. Femoral large bore sheath management: how to prevent vascular complications from vessel puncture to sheath removal. Circ Cardiovasc Interv. 2024;17(9):e014156.
17. Vo HV, et al. Evaluation of hemodynamic changes with ultrasound cardiac output monitoring during burn wound excision and skin grafting in severely burned patients: a prospective observational study. Int J Burns Trauma. 2025;15(1):1–10.
18. Mourot JM, et al. Complications of femoral artery catheterization in pediatric burn patients. J Burn Care Res. 2009;30(3):432–6.
19. Gigengack RK, et al. Predicting blood loss in burn excisional surgery. Burns. 2023;49(3):566–72.
20. Jolly SS, et al. Routine ultrasonography guidance for femoral vascular access for cardiac procedures: the UNIVERSAL randomized clinical trial. JAMA Cardiol. 2022;7(11):1110–8.
21. Choi YH, Lee JH, Shin JJ, et al. A revised risk analysis of stress ulcers in burn patients receiving ulcer prophylaxis. Clin Exp Emerg Med. 2015;2(4):250–5. https://doi.org/10.15441/ceem.15.076. eCollection 2015 Dec.
22. Zhou YP, Zhou ZH, Xue JZ. Burns complicated with gastrointestinal haemorrhage – an analysis of 70 cases. Burns. 1993;19(2):150–2. https://doi.org/10.1016/0305-4179(93)90040-f.
23. Tlili B, Fredj H, Mokline A, et al. Upper gastrointestinal bleeding in severely burned patients: incidence, risk factors and outcome. Ann Burns Fire Disasters. 2025;38(1):38–45. eCollection 2025 Mar.
24. Prasad JK, Thomson PD, Feller I. Gastrointestinal haemorrhage in burn patients. Burns Incl Therm Inj. 1987;13(3):194–7. https://doi.org/10.1016/0305-4179(87)90165-3.
25. Kantak NA, Mistry R, Halvorson EG. A review of negative-pressure wound therapy in the management of burn wounds. Burns. 2016;42(8):1623–33. https://doi.org/10.1016/j.burns.2016.06.011. Epub 2016 Jul 1.
26. Megahed MA, El-Helbawy RH, Gad SS, et al. Base deficit, serum albumin level and blood haemoglobin concentration can be used as predictor factors for mortality in major burn patients. Ann Burns Fire Disasters. 2020;33(3):209–15.
27. Kenworthy P, Grisbrook TL, Phillips M, et al. Bioimpedance spectroscopy: a technique to monitor interventions for swelling in minor burns. Burns. 2017;43(8):1725–35.
28. Palmieri TL. Transfusion and infections in the burn patient. Surg Infect. 2021;22(1):49–53.
29. Li XJ, Tang WB. Pay attention to persistent inflammation-immunosuppression-catabolism syndrome in the late stage of severe burns. Zhonghua Shao Shang Yu Chuang Mian Xiu Fu Za Zhi. 2023;39(5):407–10.
30. Torres CM, Kenzik KM, Saillant NN, et al. Timing to first whole blood transfusion and survival following severe hemorrhage in trauma patients. JAMA Surg. 2024;159(4):374–81.

Chapter 5
New Measures for Inhalation Injury Management

Chuanan Shen, Wei Liu, and Ting He

Burns to head and face are often combined with inhalation injuries, which constitute a complex trauma to the trachea and lung parenchyma caused by exposure to heat and/or toxic smoke [1]. Thermal injuries primarily affect the tracheal lumen, while toxic smoke can damage the bronchioles and alveoli. The combination of thermal and toxic smoke injuries complicates the clinical picture, particularly when extensive surface burns are present alongside inhalation injuries. Such cases are associated with a mortality rate exceeding 50%, necessitating meticulous medical attention and intervention.

The two causative factors result in intricate pathophysiological changes, including thermal injuries to the upper respiratory tract, chemical injuries to the lower respiratory tract, impairment to lung interstitium, and toxicity into the whole circulation [2]. Consequently, there is a significant increase in sputum and necrotic mucus, causing tracheal edema, bleeding, ulceration, spasm, and potential obstruction. These conditions can further lead to complications such as pneumonia, pulmonary edema, atelectasis, pulmonary infection, and even acute respiratory distress syndrome (ARDS) [3].

Based on our clinical experience, we have developed a targeted and comprehensive care approach for the diagnosis and treatment of inhalation injuries. This approach has demonstrated satisfactory outcomes in practical clinical applications, effectively addressing the complexities associated with these injuries.

C. Shen (✉) · W. Liu · T. He
The Medical Department of Burn and Plastic Surgery, The 4th Medical Center, PLAGH, Beijing, China

C. Shen (ed.), *Novel Strategies for Critical Burn Care*,
https://doi.org/10.1007/978-981-92-0325-3_5

5.1 Diagnosis

5.1.1 New Thinking on Diagnosis

Accurate and comprehensive diagnosis of inhalation injury in the early stages post-burn is pivotal. We advocate for a diagnostic approach characterized by "being joint, dynamic, comprehensive and specialized," aiming to lay the groundwork for precise treatment strategies. This principle emphasizes a two-pronged approach of combining best practices in burn care for treating body surface wounds and insights from respiratory medicine for addressing respiratory mucus and lung tissue repair.

[Joint Diagnosis]
The diagnostic process should consider the patient's history, symptoms and physical signs, findings from fiberoptic bronchoscopy, laboratory tests, imaging studies, and other relevant examinations.

1. **Patient History**. Thorough documentation of the circumstances surrounding the injury, including whether it occurred in a confined space, exposure to flames or smoke, presence of burns or smoke inhalation, and behaviors like running or crying for help.
2. **Symptoms and signs. Symptoms:** ① chest tightness, suffocation, and dyspnea; ② sore throat, hoarseness, and dysphagia; ③ wheezing and irritating cough; and ④ irritability and coma. **Signs:** ① burns to the head and face; ② scorched nose hair, and a large amount of charred substance in the mouth and nose; and ③ elevated respiratory rate and auscultatory findings of lung rales.
3. **Laboratory tests**. Among the various parameters of arterial blood gas analysis, pH, partial pressure of carbon dioxide (pCO_2) and oxygen (PaO_2), oxygen saturation, lactic acid, and alveolar-arterial oxygen partial pressure difference ($AaDO_2$) are helpful to evaluate the patient condition and prognosis. The oxygenation index (PaO_2/FiO_2) serves as an important indicator for hypoxia, reflective of acute lung injury or respiratory failure.
4. **Fiberoptic bronchoscopy.** This diagnostic tool complements the initial assessment by providing direct visualization of airway injuries. For high-risk patients, fiberoptic bronchoscopy is utilized for diagnosis confirmation and allows for precise evaluation of the depth, extent, and location of injuries. In the early stage post-inhalation injury, erythema, congestion, edema and erosion of airway mucosa, and carbon deposition could be seen under the fiberoptic bronchoscopy.
5. **Imaging examination**. Chest X-ray and CT scans play a vital role in diagnosing inhalation injuries and assessing the patient's condition by providing information on lung injury severity, infections, and areas of atelectasis.

[Dynamic Diagnosis]
Frequent inspection (twice daily) of airway mucosa shedding, charred substance removal, and mucosa healing status is necessary for the evaluation of severity of

inhalation injury at different stages. Continuous evaluation of mucosal burn depth, typically on a weekly basis, allows for timely updates to the diagnosis to mitigate risks of airway complications such as contracture or stenosis. With the progress of treatment, the presence of charred particles would gradually decrease, the mucosa shedding and pseudomembrane increase, bleeding, mucosal congestion and edema gradually decrease, and the sputum become thinner in density and lighter in color.

[Comprehensive Diagnosis]
Patient history is carefully reviewed to assess potential smoke-related injuries. Patients with tracheotomy can be examined with fiberoptic bronchoscope to determine the depth of tracheal and bronchial injuries, and with electronic laryngoscope to observe injuries in the oral, nasal, and throat regions, including potential vocal cord damage. Imaging studies and ultrasound examinations aid in identifying injuries and alterations in alveoli, bronchioles, and other lung tissues at various levels. A comprehensive diagnosis of both the upper and lower respiratory tracts is crucial to avoid overlooking any potential injuries.

[Respiratory Specialist Consultation]
Given the dynamic nature of the patient's condition, continuous changes necessitate the expertise of respiratory specialists who are adept at discerning subtle respiratory abnormalities and possess specialized knowledge in diagnosing and treating respiratory disorders. Consultations with respiratory specialists are recommended to leverage their expertise. However, it is also essential to critically assess their recommendations, as inhalation injuries entail complexities beyond typical pneumonia, representing a multifaceted injury with mucosal injuries. Tailored and personalized treatment plans should be developed based on the individual patient's circumstances.

5.1.2 Severity Classification

The classification system currently used in China employs a three-grade method to assess the severity of inhalation injuries: Injuries above the glottis are categorized as mild, those above the tracheal carina as moderate, and those below the tracheal carina as severe [4].

Inhalation injury involves burns to special structures, necessitating a nuanced evaluation of airway injury severity from a wound assessment perspective. Therefore, in addition to considering the location and extent of the injury, the depth of the injury must be carefully evaluated when devising an optimal treatment strategy.

Based on our experience, we propose a classification system for inhalation injuries that considers the burn depths of airway mucosa:

Degree I (Mild): limited areas of erythema, mild hyperemia, and edema of airway mucosa; focal charred debris deposition; no airway obstruction; healing expected

Table 5.1 Classification of severity of inhalation injury

Severity	Mild	Moderate	Severe
Areas affected	Supraglottic	Above tracheal carina	Below tracheal carina
Mucosal burn depth	Degree I	Degree II	Degree III
Smoke inhalation	No	No	Yes

within approximately 7 days; and favorable prognosis without scarring or airway contracture

Degree II (Moderate): patchy erythematous areas with significant hyperemia and edema; patchy ulcerative lesions and pseudomembrane; wider carbon deposition in the trachea and bronchi; bleeding from the wound surface; no airway obstruction; healing expected within 10–14 days; and possible stripes of scar formation in later stages

Degree III (Severe): erosion and bleeding of airway mucosa; luminal swelling and constriction; extensive mucosal necrosis; 5 ~ 7 days post-injury, necrotic tissue may slough off or expose cartilage; wound bed bleeding; various degrees of airway stenosis, collapse or obstruction; healing unlikely within 14 days; and potential scars and stenosis formation in later stages

Additionally, in cases where patients present with a clear history of smoke inhalation supported by relevant imaging findings, it is recommended to consider a diagnosis of severe inhalation injury, even in the absence of apparent airway injury observed during bronchoscopy.

In this way, a comprehensive classification system that incorporates burn extent, burn depths, and the presence of smoke inhalation injury has been established (Table 5.1), with the aim of supporting optimal treatment strategies.

5.2 Treatment

5.2.1 Early Stage Emergency Care

In the initial stages following inhalation injury, adherence to strict tracheotomy indications is paramount. When emergency tracheotomy is not warranted, maintaining clear airways and reducing airway edema are crucial [5]. Recommended treatment measures include:

1. **Patient Positioning:** placing the patient in a sitting or semi-sitting position.
2. **Medication Administration:**
    - Administering low-dose dexamethasone sodium phosphate injection (10 mg) to alleviate edema
    - Using mannitol injection (125 mL) and furosemide injection (20 mg) to promote dehydration and diuresis

3. **Fluid Management:** ensuring appropriate fluid infusion
4. **Oxygen Therapy:** employing nasal tubing or masks for oxygen delivery
5. **Aerosol Therapy:** enhancing aerosol therapy to mitigate airway swelling and reduce obstruction risks

However, endotracheal intubation or tracheotomy is warranted in cases of excessive respiratory secretions, gastric reflux and bleeding, or persistent hypoxemia unresponsive to oxygen delivery via nasal tubing or mask.

5.2.2 *Airway Management [6]*

I. **Aerosol therapy**

Aerosol therapy, a critical component of inhalation injury management, aims to reduce local respiratory tract inflammation, bronchiectasis, and sputum viscosity and enhance airway mucosa healing. Common aerosol therapy regimens include:

① For severe inhalation injury, a compound solution of 5 mg of dexamethasone, 15 mg of ambroxol, 15 mL of recombinant human epidermal growth factor, and 8 U of chymotrypsin in 100 mL of sterilized water is used once every 4 h. Dexamethasone should be discontinued after 3 days of use.

② For mild and moderate inhalation injury, 3 mL of acetylcysteine solution for inhalation use and 4 mL of budesonide suspension for inhalation use in 2 mL of sterile water are given once every 8 h, and 2 mL of ipratropium bromide solution for inhalation and 2.5 mL of salbutamol sulfate solution for inhalation use in 2 mL of sterile water are given once every 8 h.

③ For patients in the recovery phase, a compound solution of 2 mL of ipratropium bromide solution for inhalation use and 2.5 mL of salbutamol sulfate solution for inhalation use and 3 mL of acetylcysteine solution for inhalation use once is given once every 8 h.

In addition to the common aerosol therapy regimens, patients with airway mucosal bleeding can be given 6 U pituitrin in 3 mL 0.9% sodium chloride solution once every 8 h; patients with thick sputum can be given a large dose of ambroxol (300 mg) at the rate of 4 mL/h intravenously. Airway hyperresponsiveness can be treated with 0.25 g aminophylline in 5% glucose solution (48 mL) at the rate 5 mL/h or 0.25 g dihydroxypropyl theophylline intravenously.

II. **Expectoration in prone position**

Essential for airway clearance, expectoration involves suctioning phlegm and necrotic tissue from the mouth, nasal cavity, and airways. Postural drainage aids in removing deeper lung secretions. For patients with extensive burns and inhalation injuries, expectoration can be facilitated through chest percussion, either manual or mechanical, and postural drainage [7]. For patients with pulmonary infections requiring intensive drainage and expectoration, prolonged prone positioning is frequently employed. If a patient experiences discomfort in the prone position, reducing the duration of each prone session while increasing the frequency of roll-overs is recommended to ensure an extended total time spent in the prone position.

The prone positioning protocol may vary based on the patient's condition:

① Early stage (1 ~ 2 days post-injury): 1 h prone position followed by 2 h supine, with 8 rollovers per day
② Transition stage (3 ~ 4 days post-injury): 2 h prone followed by 2 h supine, with 6 rollovers per day
③ Adaptation stage (5 ~ 7 post-injury): 2 h prone followed by 1 h supine, with 8 rollovers per day
④ Later stage: Adjust prone positioning duration and rollover frequency based on individual patient needs, maintaining a minimum 2:1 prone-to-supine ratio.

III. **High-concentration oxygen therapy at normal air pressure**

Studies have shown that hyperbaric oxygen treatment can elevate a patient's arterial oxygen partial pressure to 1150 mmHg, enhancing oxygen diffusion into tissues, increasing tissue oxygen content, and correcting airway cell hypoxia to facilitate airway repair [8]. However, this treatment is often impractical for patients with extensive burns, and inhalation injuries for the facilities in the hyperbaric oxygen chamber are quite limited to support patients in critical conditions.

High-concentration oxygen therapy at normal pressure can achieve an arterial oxygen partial pressure of 300 mmHg, also enhancing tissue oxygen content. In clinical practice, we administer 100% pure oxygen at normal pressure to burn patients for 30-min sessions, 1–3 times a day. This approach has demonstrated efficacy in promoting tissue repair while mitigating the risk of oxygen toxicity associated with prolonged high-concentration oxygen therapy.

IV. **Fiberoptic bronchoscope therapy**

Fiberoptic bronchoscopy aids burn specialists in visualizing the extent and locations of respiratory mucosal injuries, clearing airway secretions and necrotic tissue, sampling from deeper lung areas, and administering medications [9]. Similar to changing wound dressings on the skin, the frequency of fiberoptic bronchoscope use is tailored to the severity of airway mucosal injury.

The updated 2019 Guide on Application of Adult Diagnostic Flexible Bronchoscopy in China has removed airway lavage operations and made it permissible to identify and manage bleeding sites using fiberoptic bronchoscopy in post-tracheotomy patients experiencing significant hemoptysis. Patients with severe inhalation injuries are prone to respiratory tract bleeding, particularly during mucosal exfoliation and repair phases. Local medications can be applied under fiberoptic bronchoscopy to address bleeding in the following forms of combinations: ① 6 U pituitrin +20 mL 0.9% sodium chloride solution, ② 1 mg adrenaline hydrochloride solution +20 mL 0.9% sodium chloride solution, and ③ 1 U Haemocoagulase Agkistrodon(HCA) +10 mL 0.9% sodium chloride solution.

XXII. **Artificial nose**

For patients with cuffed tracheostomy tubes, where airflow bypasses the nose's natural warming, humidifying, and filtering functions, significant moisture loss (800–1000 mL/day) occurs through the artificial airway. Inadequately humidified inspired air can lead to thickened or encrusted secretions, mucous plugging, and severe complications like pneumonia and atelectasis. To optimize airway and secretion management, heat and moisture exchangers (HMEs), also known as artificial noses, can be utilized [10]. These passive humidifiers warm, humidify, and filter inspired air (Fig. 5.1). Artificial noses are recommended in the scenario where the patient, given continuous low oxygen flows (3-5 L/min), does not experience any breath difficulties and has oxygen saturation (SaO_2) levels between 96% and 100% and arterial oxygen partial pressure (PaO2) exceeding 83 mmHg.

VI. **High-flow humidifier**

While the artificial nose offers a simple and cost-effective solution, it may not suffice for patients with dehydrated airways. In such cases, the high-flow humidifier, an advanced electronic counterpart to the artificial nose, provides enhanced support.

The high-flow humidifier is a sophisticated, adjustable device equipped with a built-in humidification and heating system [11]. It delivers air at 100% relative humidity (44 mgH2O/L) and a temperature of 37 °C, with a flow rate ranging from 2 to 60 L/min and adjustable oxygen concentrations between 21% and 100% (Fig. 5.2). Additionally, it features an integrated oxygen concentration monitor that offers real-time feedback on flow, temperature, and oxygen levels. This apparatus optimizes care by delivering positive-pressure support, dynamically regulating air temperature and humidity, adjusting flow rates as needed, and effectively alleviating dyspnea in patients.

By enhancing airway humidification, promoting secretion drainage, preventing encrusted secretions, reducing choking and pneumonia risks, and improving PaO_2 and SaO_2, the high-flow humidifier significantly benefits patients. The airway humidification volume is typically adjusted dynamically based on sputum

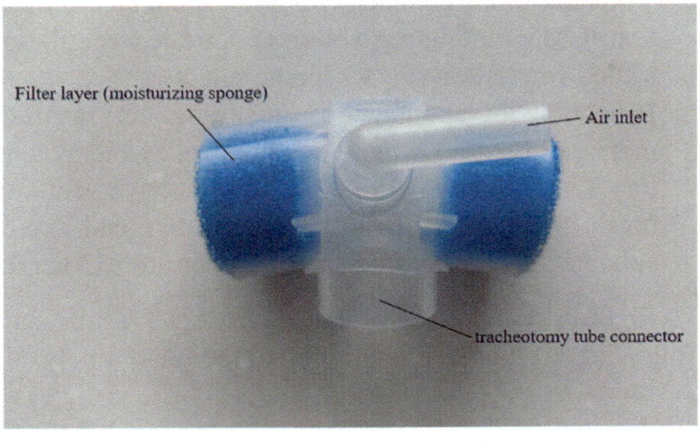

Fig. 5.1 Artificial nose

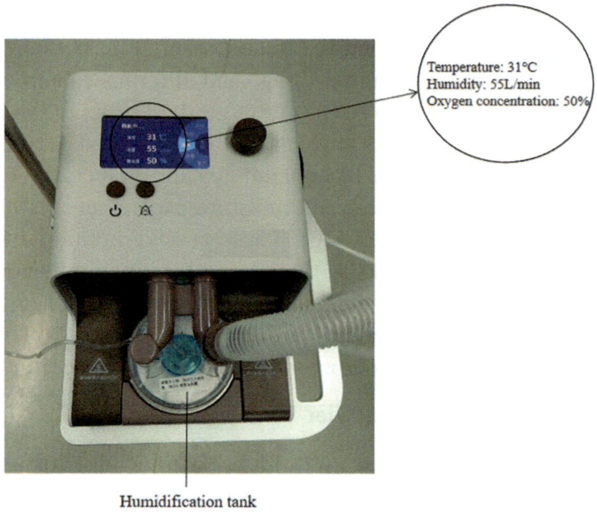

Fig. 5.2 High-flow humidifier

viscosity, ranging from 35 to 40 L/min to 60 to 70 L/min, with the temperature set at 37 °C and oxygen concentration tailored to arterial blood gas (ABG) results.

5.2.3 Respiratory Management

I. **Mechanical ventilation**

In patients with inhalation injuries experiencing progressive dyspnea due to atelectasis and pneumonia, mechanical ventilation can be employed to enhance gas exchange, optimize patient comfort, and expedite the recovery of spontaneous breathing [12]. Various mechanical ventilation modes are utilized based on the severity of inhalation injuries:

① For unconscious patients with weak spontaneous breathing, control mode ventilation (CMV) including volume controlled ventilation (VCV) and pressure controlled ventilation (PCV) can be selected.

② Patients with spontaneous breathing but insufficient respiratory effort and increased breath frequency may benefit from synchronized intermittent mandatory ventilation (SIMV) for lung-protective ventilation, involving low tidal volumes (4–7 mL/kg), appropriate positive end expiratory pressure (PEEP), and suitable airway pressure (plateau pressure $\leq$ 30 cmH2O).

Rigorous monitoring of vital signs, ABG results, and laboratory tests is essential following mechanical ventilation to facilitate timely adjustments.

II. **Extracorporeal membrane oxygenation (ECMO)**

In cases of severe inhalation injury complicated by acute respiratory distress syndrome, respiratory failure, ventilation-diffusion disorders, or refractory hypoxemia despite conventional interventions, including prone-position ventilation, high-frequency oscillatory ventilation, and lung-protective strategies, consideration should be given to extracorporeal membrane oxygenation (ECMO) for advanced respiratory support [13]. If a patient exhibits persistent hypoxemia with a PaO_2/FiO_2 ratio below 100 mmHg and a respiratory rate exceeding 35 breaths per minute, ECMO may be warranted.

5.2.4 Sedation and Analgesia

To address pain and ensure patient comfort during mechanical ventilation, appropriate sedation and analgesia regimens are essential. Options include:

- Tramadol hydrochloride sustained-release tablets (0.1 g) or flurbiprofen axetil injection solution (50 mg)
- If initial choices are ineffective, dexmedetomidine hydrochloride solution for injection (200 μg) and 48 mL of 0.9% sodium chloride solution for injection with their load dose and maintenance dose being adjusted based on patient weight, given through a continuous infusion pump, can be considered.
- For shallow, rapid breathing or noticeable patient-ventilator mismatches but with stable blood pressure, continuous infusion of 0.5 g propofol at 3–15 mL/h is recommended. Alternatively, continuous infusion of 4 mg Remifentanil with 50 mL 0.9% sodium chloride solution at 2 mL/h can be considered. In case of inadequate response, propofol may be substituted with 50 mg midazolam injection solution and 50 mL 0.9% sodium chloride solution at 3 mL/h via continuous infusion pump.

5.2.5 Anti-infection Therapy

It is reported that the mortality of burn patients is 20% higher when combined with inhalation injury and 60% higher with pneumonia [14]. Therefore, strict adherence to sterile techniques is imperative for those with extensive burns and inhalation injuries. Monitoring of body temperature, respiratory rate, regular phlegm cultures, and key infection indicators like white blood cell count (WBC), procalcitonin (PCT), and C-reactive protein (CRP) levels is crucial. Initial broad-spectrum antibiotics should be followed by targeted antibiotics based on phlegm culture results.

5.2.6 *Treatment of Burn Wounds*

For patients with large burns, the wounds give rise to all possible complications. Therefore, the core of burn treatment is to achieve wound closure and healing as soon as possible. However, if inhalation injury leads to pulmonary inflammation or infection, impacting respiratory function and oxygenation, the feasibility of general anesthesia must be carefully evaluated. Surgical procedures should be postponed in the presence of complications such as atelectasis, pulmonary infections, acute respiratory distress syndrome (ARDS), or respiratory failure until pulmonary conditions improve.

[Typical Case]

Case 1

The patient, male, aged 38 years, sustained multiple flame burns following an E-motorcycle battery deflagration incident. The patient was startled from sleep by thick smoke, then ran, and shouted for help. He arrived at our center 7 h postburn and complained of chest tightness, suffocation, sore throat, hoarseness, constant cough, expectoration, and other discomfort.

Physical examination: The patient was conscious. Lung auscultation found noisy breath sounds in both lungs, with slightly lower pitched sounds in the left lung. Vital signs: body temperature, 36 °C; pulse, 124 bpm; blood pressure, 170 mmHg/87 mmHg; respiratory rate, 36 bpm; and SaO_2, 96%. Burn wounds could be seen on the head, face, neck, trunk, and limbs, with a total size of about 50% TBSA. The wound surface of the head, face, and neck was pale or red-and-white, with evident edema. The patient's nose hair had been scorched. His mouth was semirigid like a fish mouth, oropharynx was red and swollen, and voice was hoarse with a large amount of carbon residue on the tongue and the posterior pharyngeal wall. Most of the rotten skin of the wounds on trunk and limbs had fallen off, the wound bases on head and face, upper limbs and left lower limb were pale with diminished tenderness, and the distal parts of limbs were cold. ABG results: PaO_2, 85 mmHg and FiO_2, 33% (oxygen delivered through a nasal catheter at a flow rate of 4 L/min). Based on this, he was given tracheotomy, chest X-ray examination, and fiberoptic bronchoscopy to check the respiratory tract injuries.

Admission Diagnoses: ① burn size, 50% TBSA; burn depth, deep II degree (27%) and III degree (23%) and ② severe inhalation injury

Treatment Course: After admission, the patient was given a respiratory filter which provided oxygen at the rate of 5 L/min. Then a large amount of sputum containing charred substances was suctioned out through the mouth, nose, and the tracheal opening. Gradually, the patient developed dyspnea with increased respiratory rate and decreased SaO_2 (90%). Then he was given ventilation in SIMV mode with tidal volume of 620 mL and oxygen concentration ranging from 45% to 70%; with this his SaO_2 gradually rose to 100%.

An enhanced aerosol therapy regimen was formulated. To promote expectorant, the combination of 2 mL sterile water for injection +3 mL acetylcysteine solution for inhalation +4 mL budesonide suspension for inhalation was given every 8 h, and to restore bronchodilation, the combination of 2 mL sterile water for injection +2 mL ipratropium bromide solution for inhalation +2.5 mL salbutamol sulfate solution for inhalation was given every 8 h. Expectoration in prone position was strengthened. The patient was placed on a rollover bed, and the time in the prone position gradually increased to 4 h (prone: supine = 4:1). Phlegm was suctioned step by step, section by section.

In the first week post-injury, daily chest X-ray (Figs. 5.3 and 5.5), fiberoptic bronchoscopy (Figs. 5.4 and 5.6), and phlegm suction were performed, as well as local application of RhEGF for mucosal healing alongside dynamic assessment of respiratory tract injury. During this period, the ventilator parameters were gradually adjusted, and the oxygen concentration was gradually reduced from 70% to 35%. The airway was intermittently humidified with a high-flow respiratory humidifier, and the secretion was fully drained. Smooth breath for the patient was ensured, and SaO_2 was maintained between 98% and 100%. On the 12th day post-injury, the ventilator was removed, with continued use of the high-flow respiratory humidifier.

Given the patient's severe inhalation injury, compromised oxygenation index, and impaired pulmonary function, the risk associated with anesthesia and surgical interventions was deemed significant. Consequently, a conservative approach was adopted for managing deep burn wounds in the initial post-injury phase. With subsequent improvements noted in the patient's airway and cardiopulmonary function, the first operation of excision and grafting was scheduled for the 10th day post-injury. The second operation of excision and grafting was performed on the 19th

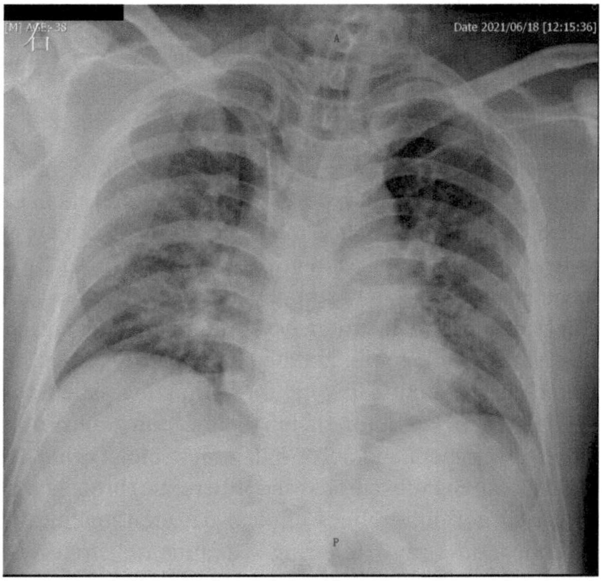

Fig. 5.3 On the day of injury, the chest X-ray examination revealed non-aggravated bilateral hilar shadows, patchy fuzzy shadows, and bilateral lung inflammation

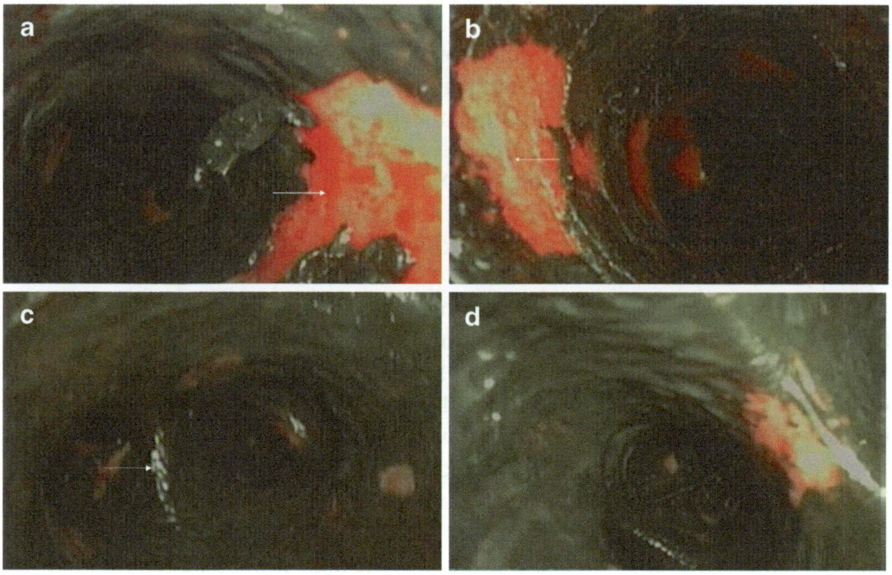

Fig. 5.4 Bronchoscopy on the day of injury. (**a**) Left main bronchus. (**b**) Right main bronchus. (**c**, **d**). Lobar bronchi. The white arrow indicates the tracheal carina. The bronchial walls exhibit a chimney-like appearance, characterized by extensive deposition of charred substances. These deposits are firm in texture and present challenges for removal from the airway mucosa

day post-injury, yielding favorable healing outcomes. On the 21st day post-injury, a chest CT scan was performed, revealing local bronchiectasis and bilateral consolidation (Fig. 5.7). Bronchoscopy on the 24th day post-injury (Fig. 5.8) revealed satisfactory respiratory mucosal healing. The tracheotomy tube was removed the following day, and a nasal tubing to provide oxygen at a rate of 3 L/min was placed. The patient reported no difficulties in breathing, and the SaO_2 was maintained between 98% and 100%.

[Discussion]

Inhalation injury encompasses the damage to the respiratory tract and lung parenchyma resulting from exposure to heat and/or chemical smoke. Studies indicate a staggering 50% mortality rate among burn patients with concomitant inhalation injury. This insidious condition, often obscured by surface skin burns, unfolds through a multifaceted pathophysiological trajectory characterized by three distinct stages: respiratory insufficiency, pulmonary edema, and infection. Early stage interdisciplinary collaboration aimed at dynamic, comprehensive, and specialized diagnostic interventions is pivotal for optimizing patient outcomes.

The severity grading of inhalation injury must transcend mere mucosal injury extent assessment and delve into a meticulous evaluation of injury depth, informed by clinical manifestations and fiberoptic bronchoscopy findings. This nuanced approach not only refines clinical decision-making but also mitigates the risk of complications by tailoring treatment strategies accordingly. Fiberoptic

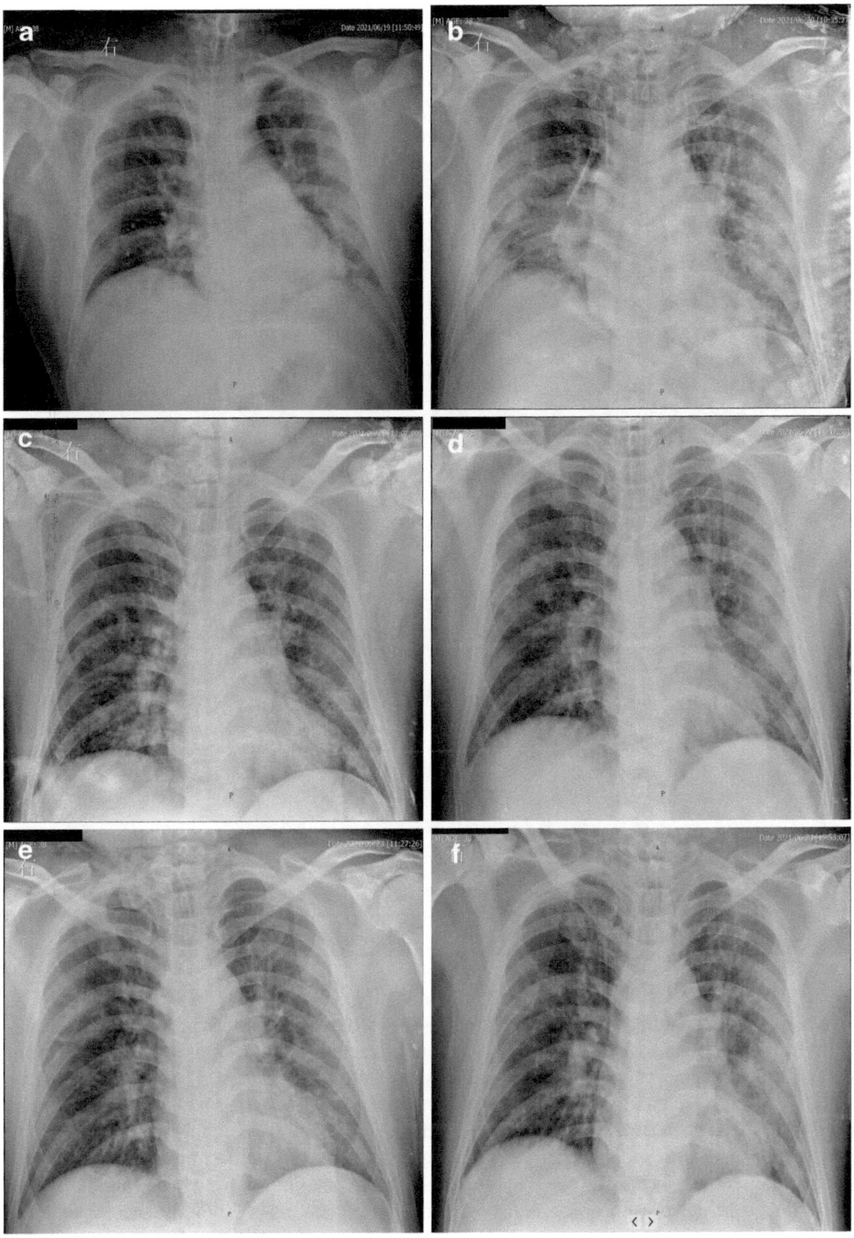

Fig. 5.5 Chest X-ray examinations in the first week post-injury. (**a**) On the first day post-injury, patchy shadows and inflammation of both lungs could be seen. (**b**) On the second day post-injury, the patchy shadows near the hilum were aggravated, with heavier shadows in the left lung. (**c**, **d**) On the third and fourth days post-injury, the shadows of both lungs obviously cleaned up. (**e**, **f**) On the fifth and sixth days post-injury, the inflammation of both lungs was relieved, the patchy shadows reduced, the texture obviously clearer, and the heart appearance smaller than before

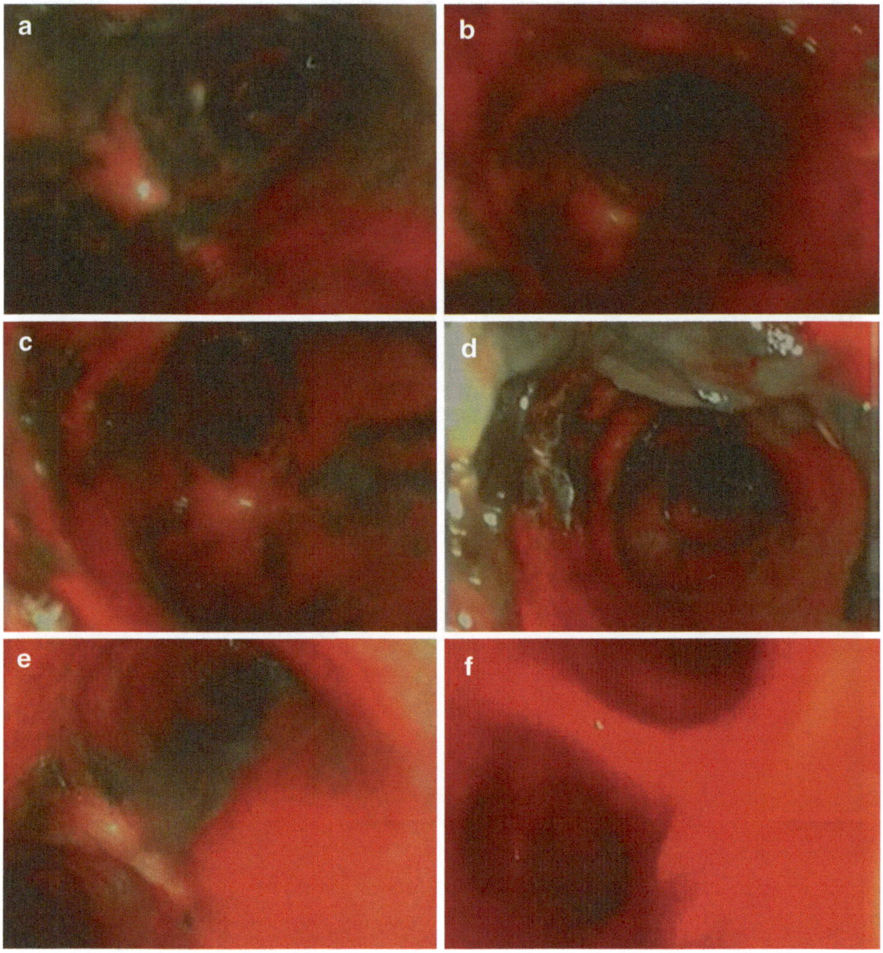

Fig. 5.6 Fiberoptic bronchoscopy 1 week post-injury. (**a**) On the first day posy-injury, exfoliation of black eschars, congestion, edema, and black viscous secretions of basal mucosa was observed. The openings of main airway branches were unobstructed without signs of stenosis. Sporadic bleeding spots were seen. (**b**) On the second day post-injury, viscous secretions could be seen in the trachea. Black eschars in the main airway branches significantly reduced, exposing congested and edematous mucosa and slightly narrowed lumen. The openings of main airway branches were unobstructed. Bleeding spots increased markedly, and black viscous secretions could be seen in secondary and tertiary bronchi. (**c, e**) On the 3rd ~ 5th day post-injury, the trachea and both left and right main bronchi were unobstructed, but with a small amount of bloody secretions and the mucosa obviously congested and edematous, covered with reduced deposition of charred substance. (**f**) On the sixth day post-injury, no black charred substances were seen in the airway. The congestion and edema of mucous membrane gradually decreased, and the secretions were mostly white and thin

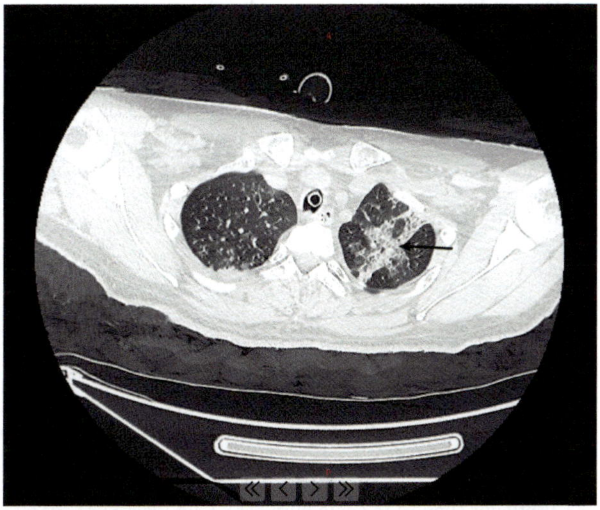

Fig. 5.7 CT examination on the 21st day post-injury revealed local bronchiectasis in both lungs. The black arrow indicates consolidation in the left lung

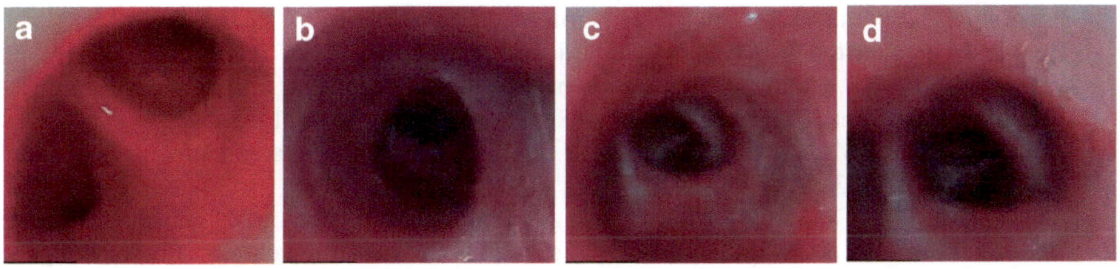

Fig. 5.8 Fiberoptic bronchoscopy on the 24th day post-injury. (a, b) Lobar bronchi. (c, d) Segmental bronchi. No congestion, edema, or bleeding of the airway mucosa was found. Each opening was unobstructed without sign of stenosis. Secretions were white and thin

bronchoscopy facilitates direct visualization of airway mucosal morphology, precise injury assessment in terms of size and depth, and monitoring of mucosal healing dynamics. Its utility extends to expeditious evaluation for tracheotomy tube removal, thereby minimizing airway exposure and lowering the likelihood of pulmonary infections. Furthermore, bronchoscopy aids in the clearance of obstructions like blood clots, secretions, eschars, and exfoliated mucosa, thereby reducing the risk of airway compromise. Additionally, it allows for sampling secretions from deeper airway recesses for bacterial culture, enhancing targeted antimicrobial therapy.

The treatment of inhalation injury mainly include ① early first aid: ensuring airway patency and alleviating airway edema, ② airway management: employing aerosol therapy to dampen local inflammatory responses, reduce bronchiectasis, enhance mucosal healing, and facilitate hemostasis; coupled with lying-position expectoration, high-concentration oxygen therapy, fiberoptic bronchoscopy interventions, and airway humidification, ③ respiratory support: utilizing mechanical ventilation, ECMO, sedation, and analgesia.

Beyond localized airway and pulmonary interventions, the holistic management of inhalation injury mandates systemic anti-infective therapy, meticulous fluid administration, wound care, nutritional optimization, psychological support, and collaboration with respiratory specialists. Given the complex nature of inhalation injury, there is a pressing need to delve deeper into diagnostic modalities and embrace a comprehensive therapeutic approach to enhance clinical outcomes.

(Chuanan Shen, Wei Liu, and Ting He)

References

1. Monteiro D, Silva I, Egipto P, Magalhães A, Filipe R, Silva A, Rodrigues A, Costa J. Inhalation injury in a burn unit: a retrospective review of prognostic factors. Ann Burns Fire Disasters. 2017;30(2):121–5.
2. Velamuri SR, Ali Y, Lanfranco J, Gupta P, Hill DM. Inhalation injury, respiratory failure, and ventilator support in acute burn care. Clin Plast Surg. 2024;51(2):221–32.
3. Bittner E, Sheridan R. Acute respiratory distress syndrome, mechanical ventilation, and inhalation injury in burn patients. Surg Clin North Am. 2023;103(3):439–51.
4. Burn and Trauma Branch of Chinese Geriatrics Society, Guo F, Zhu YS, Huang J, Wu YH, Sun ZF, Xia XB, Fu XB. National experts consensus on clinical diagnosis and treatment of inhalation injury (2018 version). Zhonghua Shao Shang Za Zhi. 2018;34(11):E004.
5. Ruiz S, Puyana S, McKenney M, Hai S, Mir H. Outcomes of tracheostomy on burn inhalation injury. Eplasty. 2023;23:e43.
6. Sun D, Zhao P, Ni JY, Sun JJ, Ren YW, Wang F, Zhu LH. Effects of airway management team in the treatment of severely mass burn patients combined with inhalation injury. Zhonghua Shao Shang Za Zhi. 2018;34(6):354–9.
7. Kubo T, Osuka A, Kabata D, Kimura M, Tabira K, Ogura H. Chest physical therapy reduces pneumonia following inhalation injury. Burns. 2021;47(1):198–205.
8. Nygaard RM, Endorf FW. Hyperbaric oxygen and mortality in burns with inhalation injury: a study of the National Burn Repository. J Burn Care Res. 2021;42(5):900–4.
9. Kumana ET, Charles WN, Milton-Jones H, Agbontaen K, Soussi S, Dunn K, Davies R, Atkins J, Beynon C, Charbonney E, Gantner D, Giles J, Jones I, Martin N, Pantet O, Shelley O, Sisson A, Sokhi J, Stewart BT, Vorster T, Vizcaychipi MP, Wood F, Yarrow J, Singh S, International burns inhalation injury consortium$_*$. Evaluating inter-and intra-rater reliability in the bronchoscopic grading of burn inhalation injury: the iBRONCH-BII study. Burns. 2025;51(5):107502.
10. Kearney A, Norris K, Bertelsen C, Samad I, Cambridge M, Croft G, Peavler S, Groen C, Doyle PC, Damrose EJ. Adoption and utilization of heat and moisture exchangers (HMEs) in the tracheostomy patient. Otolaryngol Head Neck Surg. 2023;169(5):1374–81.
11. Spoletini G, Alotaibi M, Blasi F, Hill NS. Heated humidified high-flow nasal oxygen in adults: mechanisms of action and clinical implications. Chest. 2015;148(1):253–61.
12. Al Ashry HS, Mansour G, Kalil AC, Walters RW, Vivekanandan R. Incidence of ventilator associated pneumonia in burn patients with inhalation injury treated with high frequency percussive ventilation versus volume control ventilation: a systematic review. Burns. 2016;42(6):1193–200.
13. Bain AP, Garcia I, Leveno M, Akarichi C. Early extracorporeal membranous oxygenation and burn excision in severe burn and inhalation injury. Scars Burn Heal. 2024;10:20595131241302942.
14. Lu H, Li J, Quan G, Cui H. Prophylactic systemic antibiotic and systemic glucocorticoid therapy after burn inhalation injury: a report of two cases and review of literature. Cureus. 2024;16(8):e68285.

Chapter 6
New Practices on Total Enteral Nutrition

Chuanan Shen, Xinzhu Liu, and Bohan Zhang

[Background]
In patients with extensive deep burns, two primary metabolic characteristics manifest. Firstly, there is substantial nutritional depletion attributed to heightened catabolic processes, wound evaporative losses, surgical blood loss, and increased heat production [1]. Secondly, there is an escalated nutritional requirement to facilitate wound healing, support hematopoiesis, and address increased metabolic demands [2]. Following severe burn injuries, the body not only must meet its baseline physiological needs and compensate for additional expenditures resulting from wounds and surgical interventions but also necessitates an augmented nutrient supply to enable effective wound repair, leading to a significantly elevated nutritional demand. Adequate nutritional provision is paramount for optimal wound healing, bolstered immunity, and reduced susceptibility to infections [3].

At present, the strategy of nutritional support for patients with severe burns typically commences with a combination of enteral and parenteral nutrition, and then gradually transitions to total enteral nutrition (TEN) [4]. Parenteral nutrition refers to the direct infusion of nutrients into the bloodstream via a deep venous catheter, a method associated with potential complications such as hepatic dysfunction, decreased immunity and increased risks of catheter-related sepsis [5]. In contrast, enteral nutrition represents the physiological mode of nutrient intake for the body, offering a safer, cost-effective approach that preserves gastrointestinal (GI) function and mitigates disruptions to the gut microbiota [6]. We have been implementing a total enteral nutrition strategy in the management of burn patients over the past 4 years, yielding clinically favorable outcomes.

C. Shen (✉) · X. Liu · B. Zhang
The Medical Department of Burn and Plastic Surgery, The 4th Medical Center, PLAGH, Beijing, China

C. Shen (ed.), *Novel Strategies for Critical Burn Care*,
https://doi.org/10.1007/978-981-92-0325-3_6

[About the Strategy]
Part 1. TEN Strategy

- **Timing:** Immediate initiation of Total Enteral Nutrition (TEN) is strongly recommended for extensively burned patients to optimize outcomes. Early commencement is paramount. In the initial post-injury phase, oral intake of cooled boiled water at a rate of 20–50 mL per hour is advised, with a gradual introduction of semi-fluid foods like porridge, broth, fruit juice, and yogurt based on individual tolerance. Nasogastric administration of supplemental nutrient solutions should be deferred until at least 72 h post-injury.
- **Routes:** The combination of oral, nasogastric (NG), and nasoduodenal (ND) routes is pivotal for implementing TEN (Fig. 6.1). In cases of burn size exceeding 90% or compromised gastric motility, nasoduodenal tube placement may be warranted. Detailed education on oral feeding protocols and personalized dietary plans are essential to enhance patient compliance with the prescribed regimen.
- **Amount:** Estimation of the total nutrient volume for TEN can be facilitated using established formulas. We advocate for a quick reference table of nutritional volumes for severe burn scenarios (Table 6.1). The quick reference table offers reliable approximations with a 5% variance compared to intricate calculations using conventional formulas. After the shock phase, TEN initiation typically

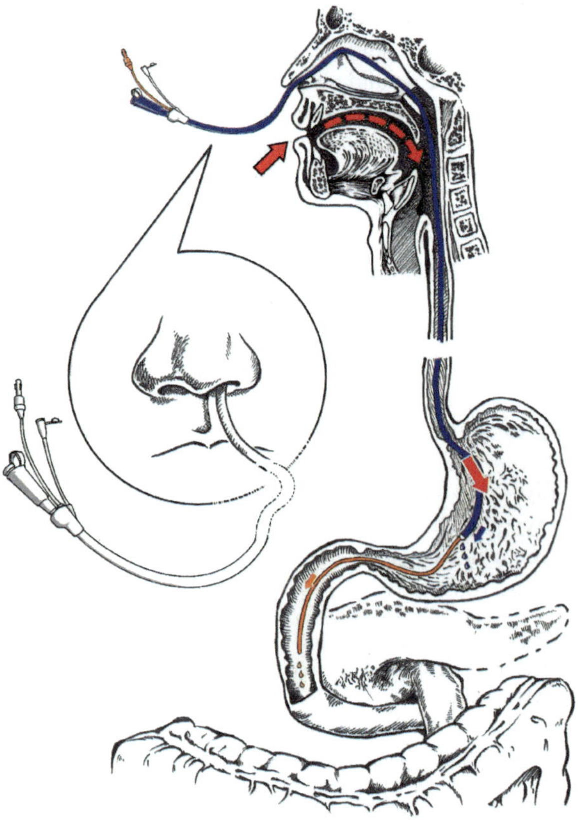

Fig. 6.1 The red arrow indicates the oral feeding route. The blue arrow, the NG route. The orange arrow, the ND route

begins at one-third of the calculated requirement, progressively escalating to full dosage, contingent on patient tolerance levels. Estimated amounts for oral intake, NG feeding and ND feeding are delineated in Table 6.2. Adjustments in feeding volumes should be based on evolving burn sizes rather than solely on the initial extent of injury.

- **Concentration, rate, and timing of enteral nutrition infusion**. During the initial stages of NG or ND feeding, the nutrition solution needs to be diluted with sterile water to 0.5 kcal/mL to avert potential diarrhea. Subsequently, the concentration can be gradually increased to 1 kcal/mL, guided by individual tolerance levels. Infusion rates should be adjusted incrementally from 50 to 150 mL/h. NG or ND feeding should be temporarily halted 1 h before and after regular meals to prevent interference with oral intake. Nutrient solutions via NG or ND routes should be administered throughout the remainder of the day.

Part 2. GI Function Protection

- **Optimal Temperature Maintenance:** The enteral nutrition solution should be maintained at 37 °C before infusion. Insulation bags are employed to preserve warmth in the solution container during infusion. Additionally, the drip line should be warmed with a heater positioned in proximity to the nostril for efficient delivery and reduced gastrointestinal tract irritation.
- **Abdominal Warmth Preservation:** Warmth in the abdominal region, particularly around the navel should be maintained. A small cotton pad or a hot water bag can be used to prevent the abdomen cooling and the resultant diarrhea.
- **Promotion of Healthy GI Microbiota:** A balanced GI microbiota is sustained through oral or nasal intake of bifidobacterium triple probiotic enteric-coated capsules, bacillus licheniformis probiotic capsules, and oral consumption of yogurt, and other probiotic-containing dairy products.

Part 3. Supporting Treatment with Blood Products

- **Addressing Anemia:** Anemia can detrimentally impact mental acuity, appetite, and intestinal function in patients, hindering the attainment of comprehensive

Table 6.1 Quick reference table for feeding amount estimation in adult burns

Burn size (% TBSA)	Quick reference (kcal)	Traditional formula (kcal)
30 ~ 49	2500	2714.15
50 ~ 69	3000	3213.80
70 ~ 89	3500	3713.44
>90	4000	4088.17

Note: The calculations were for adults weighing 70 kg and standing at 180 cm. The traditional formula commonly used in the Chinese burn community to calculate the burn patient's daily energy requirement is:
Energy requirement in kJ/d = (4184 × BSA in m^2) + (104.6 × burn size in %TBSA); BSA in m^2 = (0.0061 × height in cm) + (0.0128 × weight in kg) − 0.1529

Table 6.2 Daily feeding plan for patients with large burns

		Burn size (% TBSA)			
		30 ~ 49	50 ~ 69	70 ~ 89	≥90
Feeding amount estimation/kcal		2500	3000	3500	4000
Feeding routes	Oral/kcal	1500	1500	1500	1500
	NG/kcal	1000	1500	2000	1500
	ND/kcal				1000

Note: The remaining food after actual oral feeding is prepared into thick soups which are then fed through a nasogastric tubing. The proportion through ND feeding should be adjusted based on the patient's gastric mobility

gastrointestinal nutrition. Timely correction of anemia is imperative for optimal patient outcomes.

- **Correction of Hypoalbuminemia:** Promptly address hypoalbuminemia, which can lead to intestinal mucosal edema and diminished nutrient absorption efficiency. Corrective measures may involve plasma or albumin infusion to mitigate these adverse effects and restore optimal gastrointestinal function.

Typical Case

The patient, a 32-year-old man, sustained chemical burns all over the body from immersion in a pool containing calcium oxide and silicon dioxide at the workplace. The pool's contents reached 72 °C with a pH of 9. He was rescued promptly after 2 minutes and immediately sent to a local hospital where he received emergency treatment including tracheotomy. The patient was in critical condition and subsequently transferred to our center 23 h post-injury.

Admission diagnoses: (1) Compound burn injuries of both thermal and chemical injuries. Burn size, 100% TBSA; burn depths, deep II degree (2%TBSA), III degree (97%TBSA), IV degree (1%TBSA). (2) Acute kidney injury. (3) Hypoalbuminemia. (4) Hypocalcemia. (5) Coagulation disorder. (6) Post-tracheostomy status. (7) Hypertension.

Specialized physical examination: The patient exhibited pronounced swelling of the lips, face and neck, redness and swelling of the oral and pharyngeal areas. Extensive burns covered the entire body surface, with necrotic tissue partially sloughed, revealing a pale base. The patient reported no tenderness. His fingertips (toes) were cold. Swelling, exudation, and skin tension increased at burn sites, with secure fixation of the tracheostomy tube and bilateral subclavian venous catheters.

TEN strategy implementation: With a weight of 98 kg and height of 183 cm, the patient's daily energy requirement was 5160 kcal. Immediately after admission, a nasogastric tube was placed to gradually provide enteral nutrition. The enteral feeding started from one-third of the patient's requirement and was gradually escalated to the full capacity, based on patient tolerance. Oral nutrition began on the second day at a reduced dose of 28 kcal/300 mL to stimulate digestive function.

The NG feeding speed was controlled between 50 and 120 mL/h. The feeding was provided throughout the day with breaks around oral meals (discontinued 1 h before and after three oral meals), and continuously used for the night. Preheating nutrient solutions to 37 °C, insulating containers, and warming drip lines ensured optimal delivery. Abdominal warmth was maintained. Bifidobacterium triple probiotic enteric coated capsules and probiotic-containing dairy products such as yogurt were administered orally. Anemia and hypoalbuminemia were corrected. Blood transferrin and cholinesterase levels were monitored to evaluate the patient's nutritional status.

Clinical Progress: The patient's daily energy and protein intake through NG feeding were stable, barring surgical interventions (Fig. 6.2). The patient did not develop sepsis during the treatment course. After 39 days of treatment, the patient achieved substantial recovery, signifying successful outcomes.

Discussion

Large burns present complex challenges including critical conditions, prolonged treatment durations, potential complications, heightened energy demands, and increased nutritional needs [4]. It is generally believed that patients with large burns require supplementary parenteral nutrition. The enteral nutrition strategy we proposed and tailored for these patients emphasizes the combination of three commonly used feeding methods—oral, nasogastric (NG), and nasoduodenal (ND)—with meticulous attention to individualized care spanning supportive interventions, gastrointestinal (GI) protection, and TEN implementation.

The combination of different feeding routes confers advantages in enhancing enteral nutrition efficacy while mitigating risks complications such as fat overload syndrome, parenteral nutrition-associated liver diseases, gallbladder issues like stasis and dilation [7].

Nutritional requisites evolve throughout treatment phases, mandating dynamic assessment aligned with changing burn size for customized nutrient provision plans [8]. Continuous TEN is helpful to maintain gut health by preventing the occurrence of enterogenous sepsis and potential intestinal mucosal alterations linked to

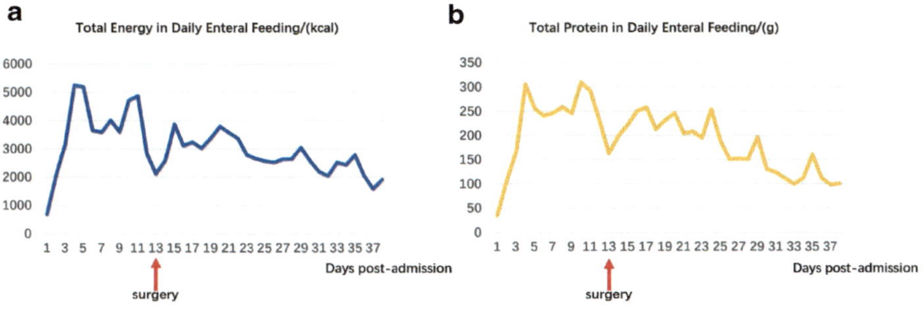

Fig. 6.2 The energy and total protein in daily enteral feeding. (**a**) The energy in daily enteral feeding; (**b**) The total protein in daily enteral feeding

prolonged parenteral nutrition use. TEN adoption reduces reliance on deep venous catheters, thereby minimizing catheter-related sepsis [9].

Undoubtedly, the successful execution of TEN is complemented by holistic patient care interventions [10]. Effective wound management curtails infection risks, addressing hypoalbuminemia alleviates intestinal edema, and rectifying anemia enhances patient consciousness, collectively fostering an environment conducive to TEN strategy implementation.

References

1. Nunez JH, Clark AT. Burn patient metabolism and nutrition. Phys Med Rehabil Clin N Am. 2023;34(4):717–31.
2. Yang YJ, et al. Effects of enteral nutrition with different energy supplies on metabolic changes and organ damage in burned rats. Burns Trauma. 2022;10:tkac042.
3. Żwierełło W, et al. Burns: classification, pathophysiology, and treatment: a review. Int J Mol Sci. 2023;24(4):3749.
4. Zhang Y, et al. Initiation of adaptive feeding within 24 h after burn injury improves nutritional therapy for severely burned patients. Front Nutr. 2024;11:1342682.
5. Fell DM, Bitetto EA, Skillman HE. Timing of enteral nutrition and parenteral nutrition in the PICU. Nutr Clin Pract. 2023;38(Suppl 2):S174–212.
6. Rousseau AF, Pantet O, Heyland DK. Nutrition after severe burn injury. Curr Opin Clin Nutr Metab Care. 2023;26(2):99–104.
7. Kano KI, et al. Strategies to maximize the benefits of evidence-based enteral nutrition: a narrative review. Nutrients. 2025;17(5):845.
8. Zagales R, et al. Optimizing nutritional needs of burn patients: an evaluation of nutritional assessment tools, feeding strategies, and their impact on patient outcomes. Am Surg. 2025;91(3):393–406.
9. Chen Y, et al. L-valine derived from the gut microbiota protects sepsis-induced intestinal injury and negatively correlates with the severity of sepsis. Front Immunol. 2024;1 5:1424332.
10. Probst S, et al. Empathy in wound care: a scoping review of its role, impact, and barriers to person-centred healing. Int Wound J. 2025;22(6):e70687.

Chapter 7
New Strategies of Plastic Surgeries for Burn Patients

Chuanan Shen, Xinzhu Liu, Jianhua Cai, and Dongjie Li

7.1 Repair of Thick Split-Thickness Graft Donor Sites with Autologous Scalp

[Background]

Large sheets of thick split-thickness skin grafts, noted for their pliability, elasticity, durability, and natural appearance attributed to the dense fibrous tissue in the dermal layer, serve as an optimal solution for wound reconstruction in aesthetically sensitive areas like hands, feet, and joints [1]. However, the harvesting process for these grafts, which extends below the dermal papilla layer, can impede donor site healing, requiring reepithelialization from residual reticular layers, hair follicles, and sweat glands, often prolonging the recovery period [2, 3]. In patients with extensive burns, harvesting large sheets of thick split-thickness grafts from areas healed from shallow burns can heighten the risk of complications such as incomplete healing, scar formation, and ulceration at the donor sites [4, 5].

Our innovative approach involves utilizing thin split-thickness autologous scalp grafts to expedite the healing of these donor sites, yielding favorable outcomes: accelerated wound closure, alleviated pain and mobility restrictions, enhanced cosmetic outcomes, and minimized scar formation. Grafting with thin split-thickness autologous scalp not only facilitates donor site healing but also enhances the quality of resurfaced skin.

[Protocol]

For patients requiring large sheets of thick split-thickness skin grafts, donor sites on the trunk or thighs are chosen, and postharvest repair is performed using thin

C. Shen (✉) · X. Liu · J. Cai · D. Li
The Medical Department of Burn and Plastic Surgery, The 4th Medical Center, PLAGH, Beijing, China

C. Shen (ed.), *Novel Strategies for Critical Burn Care*,
https://doi.org/10.1007/978-981-92-0325-3_7

split-thickness autologous scalp grafts secured with Negative Pressure Wound Therapy (NPWT) techniques.

1. **Thick Split-Thickness Skin Graft Harvest:** A large sheet of appropriately sized thick split-thickness skin grafts from the patient's trunk or thighs is harvested for the target wounds. Hemostasis at the donor site is achieved by applying gauze soaked in 1% adrenaline saline solution and adequate pressure.
2. **Thin Split-Thickness Scalp Graft Harvest:** An electric dermatome is deployed to harvest thin split-thickness grafts from the patient's scalp for repair at trunk or thigh donor sites. The harvests are carefully rinsed and then meshed. The scalp donor sites are then covered with petroleum gauze and compressed with bandages. Three days later all dressings except for the petroleum gauze were removed.
3. **Autologous Scalp Grafting:** Pieces of autologous scalp grafts should be evenly distributed at trunk or thigh donor sites. They shall not be spaced apart, but instead overlap each other at the margins with a width of about 0.5–1.5 mm. Secure fixation is ensured with mesh gauze and NPWT materials under continuous negative pressure, sealed with semipermeable biomembrane.
4. **Postoperative care:** On the seventh postoperative day, NPWT was discontinued. The grafts are carefully investigated, and dressing changes are performed until a complete healing is achieved.
5. **Precautions:** The procedure's benefits and risks should be thoroughly communicated to the patient. The thickness of the scalp grafts should be carefully controlled. The grafted autologous scalp fixation needs to be ensured to prevent dislodgement which affects the cosmetic results. NPWT is utilized to strengthen fixation and promote wound healing.

[Typical Case]

Case 7.1

The patient, a 14-year-old boy, presented with a chief complaint of hypertrophic scars on the dorsum of the left foot persisting for more than 13 years and localized refractory ulceration lasting more than 6 months. His medical history revealed the presence of a red nevus on the left foot dorsum since birth, which progressively enlarged over time. At 3 months of age, he underwent isotope therapy at a local hospital, leading to scar formation and recurrent ulceration. Prior to his referral to our facility, a recent ulceration episode failed to respond to local treatment, resulting in wound deterioration and subsequent transfer to our care.

Physical Examination: Upon evaluation, notable discrepancies in foot size were observed, with the left foot being smaller, displaying hypertrophic scars, contracture deformity, and persistent localized ulceration.

Admission Diagnoses: ① skin ulceration (0.5%TBSA with a III-degree depth) on the left foot, and ② hypertrophic scars and contracture deformity on the left foot

Treatments: After admission, debridement and grafting for the left foot, autologous thick split-thickness skin harvesting from the back (Figs. 7.1 and 7.2), and autologous scalp harvesting and grafting for the back donor site (Fig. 7.3) were

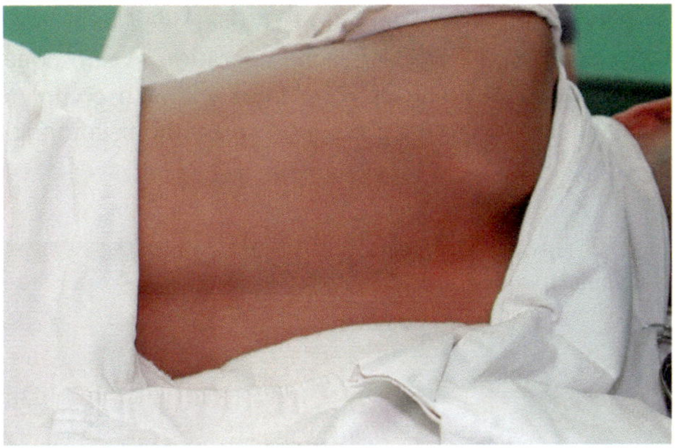

Fig. 7.1 Donor site in the back area

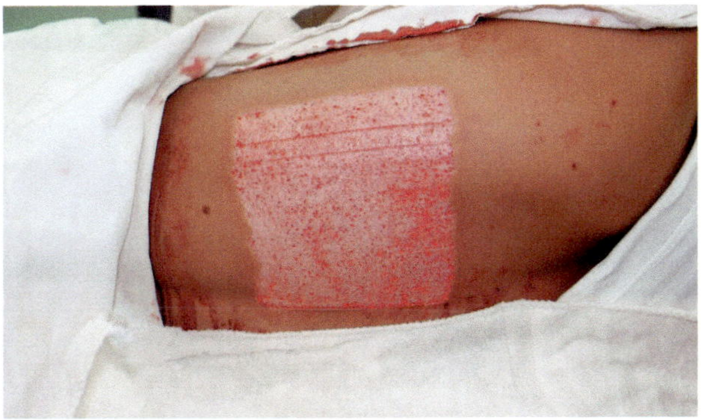

Fig. 7.2 Harvest of thick split-thickness skin graft from the back

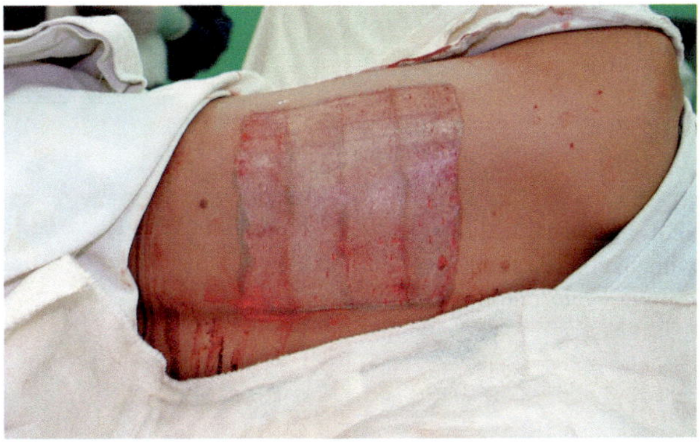

Fig. 7.3 Grafting of autologous scalp for the back donor site

performed. NPWT technique was applied to secure graft fixation (Fig. 7.4) and discontinued 7 days after the operation. A subsequent assessment revealed successful graft integration on the back with complete wound healing (Fig. 7.5), eventually exhibiting pliable skin without complications like blisters or ulcers (Fig. 7.6).

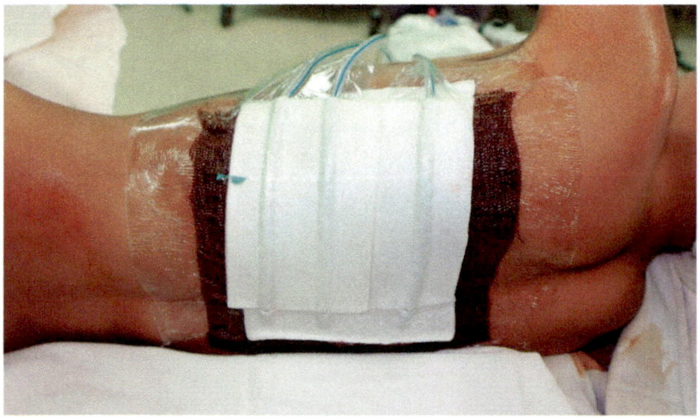

Fig. 7.4 NPWT technique was applied

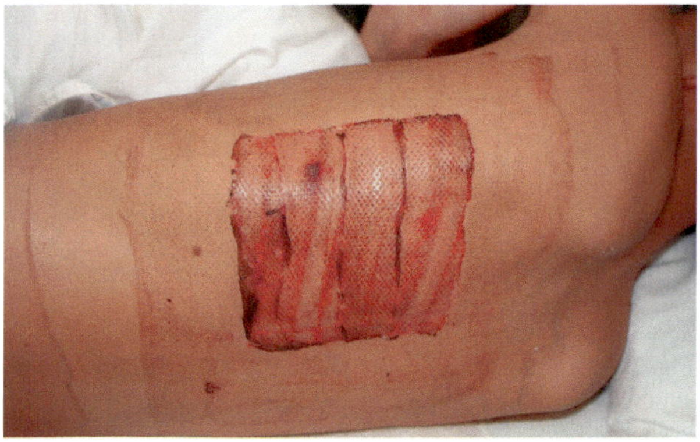

Fig. 7.5 NPWT was discontinued 7 days after operation, revealing satisfactory healing progress

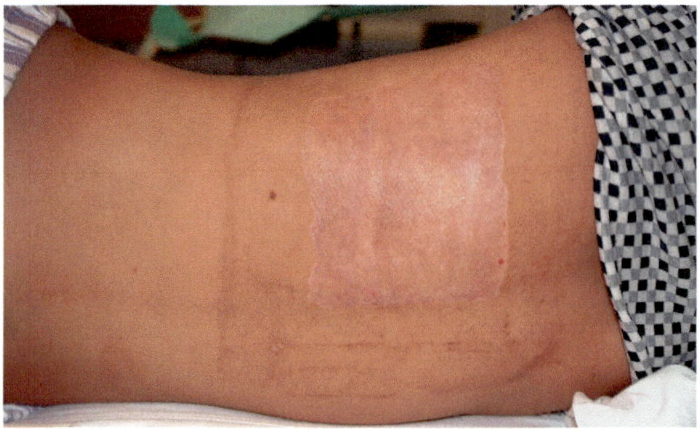

Fig. 7.6 The resurfaced skin exhibited pliable skin without complications like blisters or ulceration

Case 7.2

The patient, a 40-year-old woman, presented with a chief complaint of hypertrophic scars and contracture deformity persisting for 2 years following extensive burns. She survived burns of 92% TBSA but suffered from hypertrophic scars and contracture deformity of the healed areas, which caused both functional and cosmetic concerns. Autologous body skin sources available for plastic surgeries were in shortage. But fortunately, a significant portion of her scalp remained unaffected.

Admission Diagnoses: multiple hypertrophic scars and contracture deformity postburn.

Treatments: Surgical corrections to release neck contractures and subsequent grafting procedures were performed for the patient. Thick split-thickness skin grafts were harvested from the region healed from shallow burns on the patient's back (Figs. 7.7 and 7.8). Subsequently, the donor site was grafted with autologous scalp grafts (Fig. 7.9) and treated with NPWT (Fig. 7.10), which was dis-

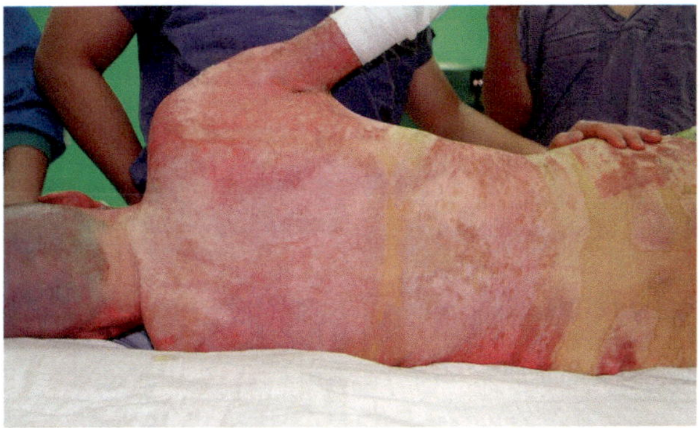

Fig. 7.7 The patient's back donor site for thick split-thickness autografts

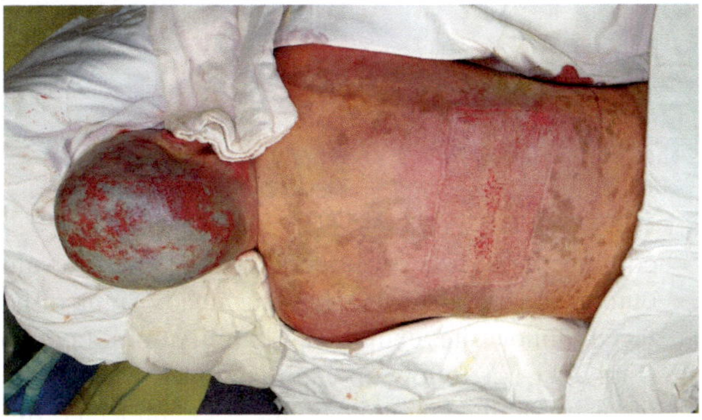

Fig. 7.8 Harvest of thick split-thickness grafts from the back and thin split-thickness grafts from the scalp

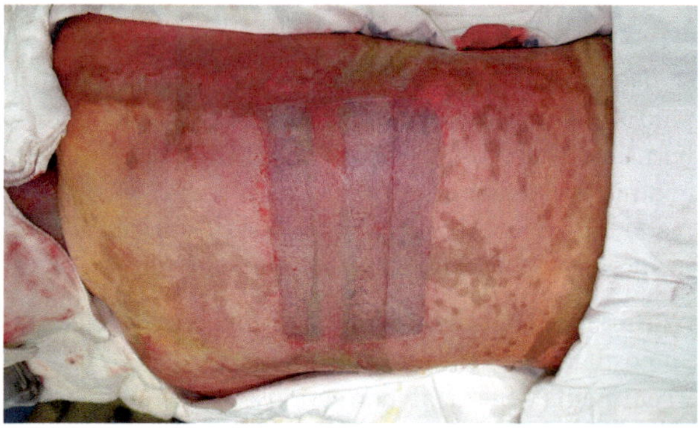

Fig. 7.9 The donor site on the back was grafted with scalp grafts

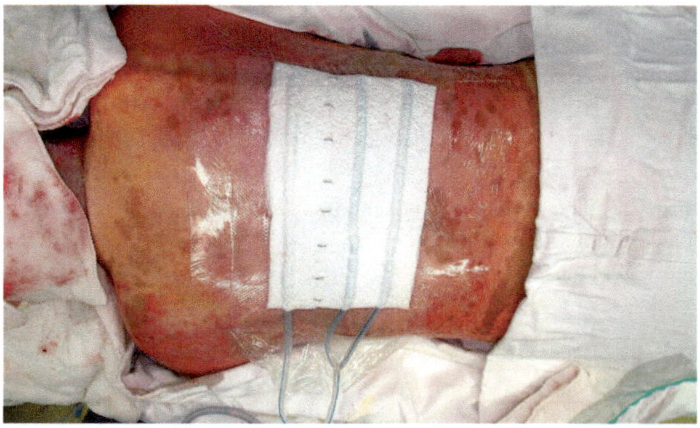

Fig. 7.10 The grafts were fixed with NPWT

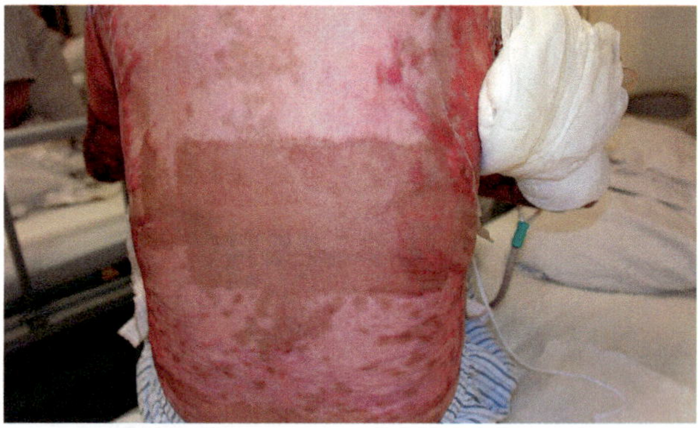

Fig. 7.11 The donor site on the back had good texture upon healing

continued 7 days postoperation. Progress evaluations revealed promising outcomes with all grafts showing steady signs of healing. Eventually, the resurfaced donor site exhibited pliability and favorable cosmetic improvements (Fig. 7.11). A follow-up examination 2 years later demonstrated a satisfactory recovery of the donor site on the back, underscoring the enduring benefits of the treatment intervention (Fig. 7.12).

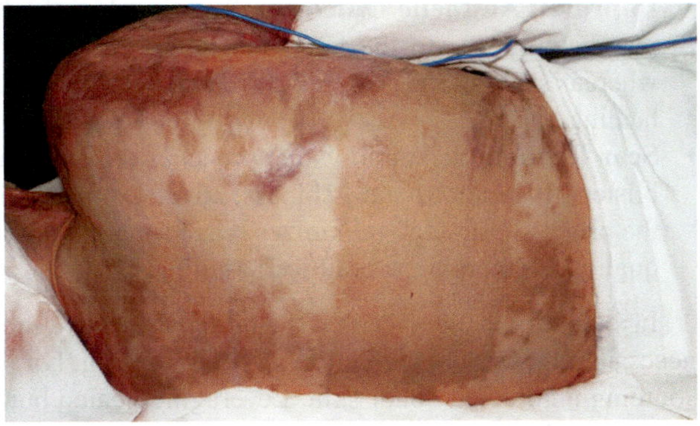

Fig. 7.12 Satisfactory functional and cosmetic results were documented in a follow-up visit 2 years later

[Discussion]

Microskin grafting, split-thickness autografts from the trunk and extremities, and scalp grafts have all been explored for repairing donor sites of thick split-thickness grafts. Though they can improve the quality of the resurfaced skin compared with the conventional methods like petroleum gauze application, they have not been widely performed. Harvesting split-thickness autografts for donor site repair introduces an additional wound of comparable size. Though donor sites of split-thickness autografts rarely develop scars, they often suffer from discoloration, posing cosmetic concerns for patients. In contrast, scalp grafts present compelling advantages such as optimal thickness, abundant hair follicles, sebaceous glands, and robust vascularity, promoting rapid healing, unhindered hair growth, and minimal scarring. Nevertheless, challenges in graft fixation on areas like the abdomen or back have historically compromised graft survival, necessitating cumbersome fixation methods like sutures or stent dressings. Addressing these challenges, the application of NPWT emerges as a simpler, more effective solution for securing these grafts, enhancing fixation outcomes.

The strategy of employing scalp grafts for repairing the thick split-thickness graft donor site offers five distinct advantages:

- **Accelerated Healing Time:** Traditional methods typically require 2–3 weeks for complete donor site healing, whereas well-fixed scalp autografts expedite healing within a mere 4 days [6].
- **Pain Alleviation:** Patients managed with traditional methods often experience significant pain during dressing changes, whereas the proposed strategy notably reduces discomfort levels since the healing process is accelerated and the frequency of dressing change is minimized [7].
- **Enhanced Mobility:** With the traditional methods, donor sites on the lower extremities would confine the patient to bed until healing, and donor sites on the back would limit the patient from supine position. In contrast, the proposed strategy incorporating NPWT allows for improved tolerance to localized pressure, enabling early mobilization postoperation without compromising the healing results [8].

- **Improved Aesthetic Outcome:** Traditional methods may lead to discoloration post-healing due to the loss of melanocytes in the epidermal germinal layer, whereas scalp grafts containing melanocytes preserve a natural appearance upon healing [9].
- **Scar Reduction:** Traditional approaches are associated with scar development, blisters, ulceration, and itchiness, adversely impacting quality of life, whereas the proposed strategy minimizes scar formation and itchiness and enhances skin quality, augmenting overall well-being [10].

In summary, patients with large burns often have scar formation and contracture necessitating surgical correction and autografting, but they often face challenges in sourcing unaffected donor skin. Leveraging healed burn wounds as donor sites for thick split-thickness autografts, which are subsequently repaired with split-thickness scalp grafts, not only ensures donor site healing but also elevates resurfaced skin quality, expanding options for scar and contracture correction surgeries.

7.2 Application of NPWT in Scar Revision Surgery

7.2.1 Tension Reduction for Incision Sites in Scar Excision Procedures

[Background]
Hypertrophic scars, particularly extensive ones, present patients with discomfort, including itching, pain, and both functional and cosmetic challenges. Some scars are prone to recurrent ulceration or non-healing, compromising the quality of life and potentially causing severe psychological distress. In pediatric cases, hypertrophic scars may impede growth and development [11–13]. Surgical correction is an effective method to reduce scars, where free skin grafting or expanded skin created with a tissue expander is commonly used. Free skin grafting, though relatively straightforward, may cause color mismatch between the recipient site and its surrounding area, while also increasing donor-site scarring. Tissue expansion offers a natural appearance but involves extended treatment durations, multiple surgeries for expander placement and removal, infection risks during injection of sterile saline solution, and an extra incision. Moreover, it results in an extra donor site at risk of developing scars that can be even larger than the target one that is to be revised. In pediatric cases, the discomfort of expansion procedures can lead to poor compliance.

Direct suture post-scar excision, a more efficient alternative approach, is limited by incision tension, potentially resulting in complications like dehiscence, widened scars, or hypertrophy. To address the problem, we have been using NPWT materials and films to redistribute tension along the incision. This method has collateral benefits such as enhanced drainage and fixation. It has been applied in scar revision for hundreds of patients in our center, yielding favorable patient outcomes.

[Protocol]

1. **Preoperative preparation**

Three to six months prior to the scar revision procedure, traction exercises on the normal skin surrounding the scar can be initiated, that is, to repeatedly apply a pulling force to the surrounding normal skin, so as to relax the skin and reduce the tension along the future incision. Preoperatively, iodophor was applied to the ulceration areas of the scar for 3 days consecutively, with the patient bathing a day before surgery. It should be noted that dirt in scar creases should be gently brushed off.

2. **Procedure implementation**

The procedure is performed under general anesthesia. For scars suitable for complete excision in a single session, the incision follows their natural contours; for scars requiring multiple sessions, an incision is made along one edge, gradually separating the scar tissue from underlying tissues until maximum tension is encountered. Where the maximum tension is encountered, a cut in the upright scar perpendicular to the surgical field surface is made. The cut's depth equals the maximum width of the scar tissue to be removed. Traction sutures are then placed at the end points of the vertical cut and its corresponding opposite edge. The two points are pulled and approximated with the traction sutures to assess tension level and determine excision width (Fig. 7.13). The extent of scar removal is premised on the successful approximation of the incision edges. During the procedure, residual scar tissue on both sides of the incision can be delicately thinned with a scalpel to ensure even and precise approximation. Electronic spring scales can gauge tension along the incision (Fig. 7.14), aiding in the selection of proper sutures.

NPWT dressings (polyvinyl alcohol) can be trimmed or spliced, so as to entirely cover the surgical site. The edges of the NPWT dressings are cushioned with an antibacterial medical dressing before applying a medical film. When applying the film, it is necessary to gently pull the skin on both sides of the incision toward the incision line to minimize tension along the line.

3. **Postoperative care**

NPWT with pressure from −40 to 20 kPa is continuously applied. The field is carefully inspected for signs of air leakage, bleeding, effusion, and odor.

In our experience, incision areas may have their dressings opened for the first time on the eighth day postoperation to monitor healing progress. Sutures can be removed intermittently or entirely contingent on healing progress, followed by the resumption of NPWT until the 14th day postoperation. Subsequently, the medical films are renewed to gently draw the skin from both sides of the incision toward the opposing side. The medical films are removed by the 16th day postoperation.

Upon complete wound healing, medical films should be applied to continuously draw the skin from both sides of the incision toward the opposite side for tension reduction over the subsequent 3 months, and the patient should be advised to wear tailored elastic garments, use scar gel pads on the incision site, and adhere to anti-scar medication regimens for the ensuing year.

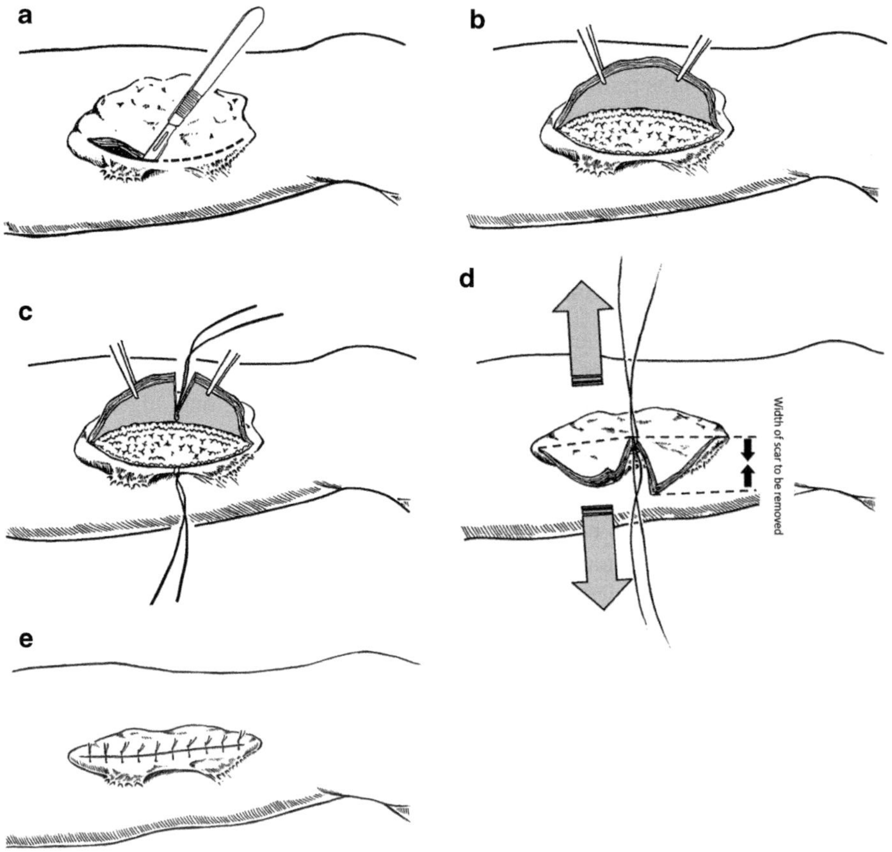

Fig. 7.13 Section-by-section scar excision. (a) An incision is made inside of the scar, along the edge on one side. (b) Scar tissue is gradually dissociated subcutaneously from this side to the opposite side. (c) A vertical cut is made to the plate where the maximum tension is encountered during scar dissociation. The depth of the cut is the maximum width of the scar tissue that is to be excised. (d) The two points are pulled and approximated with the traction sutures to help evaluate the tension and determine the width of the scar that can be excised. (e) The two edges of the remaining scar tissues are approximated and sutured

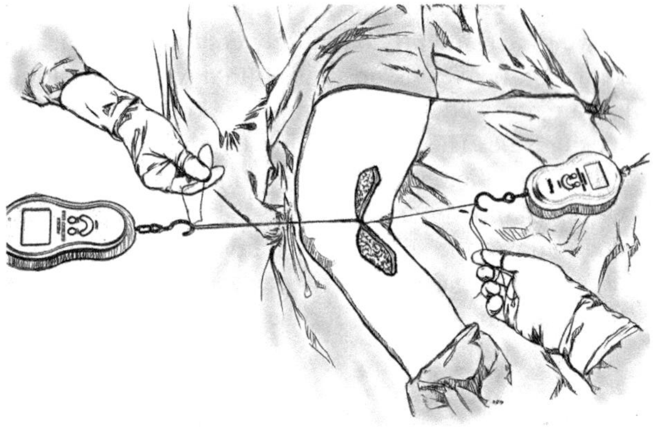

Fig. 7.14 Measurement of incision tension with spring scales

4. **Precautions**

① **Selective Scar Treatment:** Direct excision and suturing may not be suitable for all scars. A thorough preoperative assessment is essential to prevent excessive tension along the incision, which could impede suturing or compromise joint function and postoperative mobility.

② **Optimal NPWT Application:** After applying NPWT materials, two elongated strips of medical film should be placed perpendicular to the surgical incision, spaced from each other, with half of the film attached to each side of the incision and the other half gently pulled toward the opposite side to alleviate the tension along the incision (Fig. 7.15).

③ **Proper Fixation Measures:** To ensure secure fixation, the dimensions of the NPWT dressings should extend at least 3 cm beyond the sutured incision's edges. Additionally, the medical film should extend at least 5 cm beyond the outer edge of the NPWT dressings. The film size can be duly increased if excessive incision tension is encountered.

④ **Skin Protection:** The edges of NPWT dressings should be cushioned with an antibacterial medical dressing to prevent the formation of blisters on healthy skin adjacent to the negative pressure material due to shear forces.

⑤ **Timing of Subsequent Procedures:** If a second surgery is required for complete scar removal, a minimal interval of 6 months between the initial and subsequent surgeries is recommended. Additionally, traction exercises, as described in the preoperative preparation section, should be conducted for 3 to 6 months to relax the surrounding skin and alleviate tension along the future incision site.

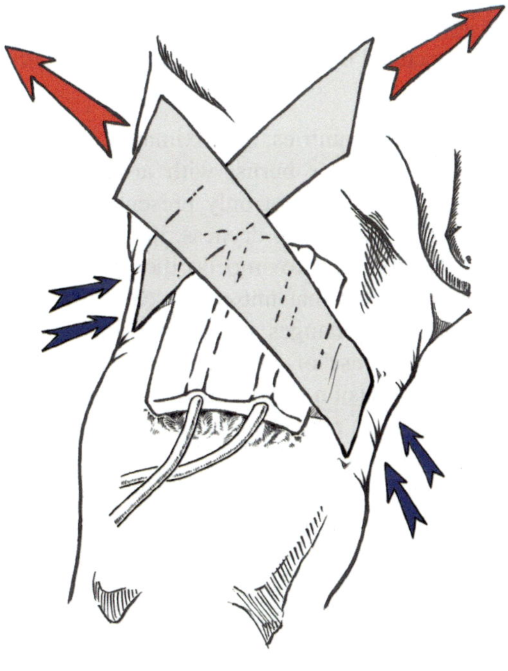

Fig. 7.15 NPWT sealing and drainage, tension reduction and fixation. The films on the two sides of the incision are pulled toward the opposite side (indicated by the red arrows), so as to relax the skin surrounding the incision. The tension along the incision is transferred to the skin at the edge of the films on both sides (indicated by the blue arrows)

[Typical Case]
The patient, a 4-year-old girl, sustained scald injury to her chest from hot water at home 1 year ago. She received dressing changes in a local hospital until wound healing was achieved. Subsequently, she gradually developed hypertrophic scars, prompting her visit to our center with main complaint of unsatisfactory scar appearance. The scar measured 35 cm^2 based on preoperative measurement. Prior to the scar excision procedure, a comprehensive evaluation using the Patient and Observer Scar Assessment Scale (POSAS) was conducted, consisting of the Observer Scar Assessment Scale (OSAS) and the Patient Scar Assessment Scale (PSAS). The OSAS enables an objective assessment of scar characteristics from a healthcare professional's perspective, focusing on parameters such as vascularity, pigmentation, thickness, relief, pliability, and surface area. Each parameter receives a score ranging from 1 to 10, aggregated to derive the final OSAS score. The PSAS captures the subjective impact of the scar on the patient's daily life, assessing aspects such as pain, itching, color, stiffness, thickness, and irregularity. Similar to OSAS, each aspect is graded on a scale of 1 to 10, culminating in the overall PSAS score. In general, higher scores indicate more severe scars with undesirable characteristics and greater impact on the patient's well-being. Pre- and post-first scar excision, the OSAS scores were 35 and 5, while the PSAS scores were 37 and 6, respectively. A second scar excision procedure was performed 6 months later, followed by suturing and application of the NPWT technique. Tensions along the incision measured 11.68 N and 12.86 N, respectively, during the two operations, and the scar areas measured 18 cm^2 and 7 cm^2, respectively, post-procedure. Both incisions healed successfully without complications like swelling or ulceration, notably, the scar area diminished by 80% after the second procedure (Fig. 7.16). Six months post the second procedure, a noticeable improvement in the affected area's appearance was observed. Pre- and post-first scar excision, the OSAS scores were 13 and 2, while the PSAS scores were 16 and 2, respectively. The favorable outcome was also acknowledged by the patient's family members.

[Discussion]
In developed countries, approximately four million people annually develop hypertrophic scars after burns, with around 70% of these cases affecting children. Hypertrophic scars not only present aesthetic and functional challenges but also give rise to issues like dryness, itching, pain, and ulceration. These complications have the potential to impede the growth and development of children. Studies [11–13] suggest that untreated scars over prolonged periods can induce adverse psychological changes in patients, including fear, depression, frustration, and a diminished sense of well-being, which even held influence on their families. As such, scar revision transcends the realm of mere medical intervention for scars; it plays a pivotal role in enhancing patient well-being within the broader scope of societal concerns.

Clinically, direct excision of large scars is rarely employed due to the substantial tension along the incision resulting from extensive tissue loss. The magnitude of skin tension plays a pivotal role in scar formation, with heightened tension

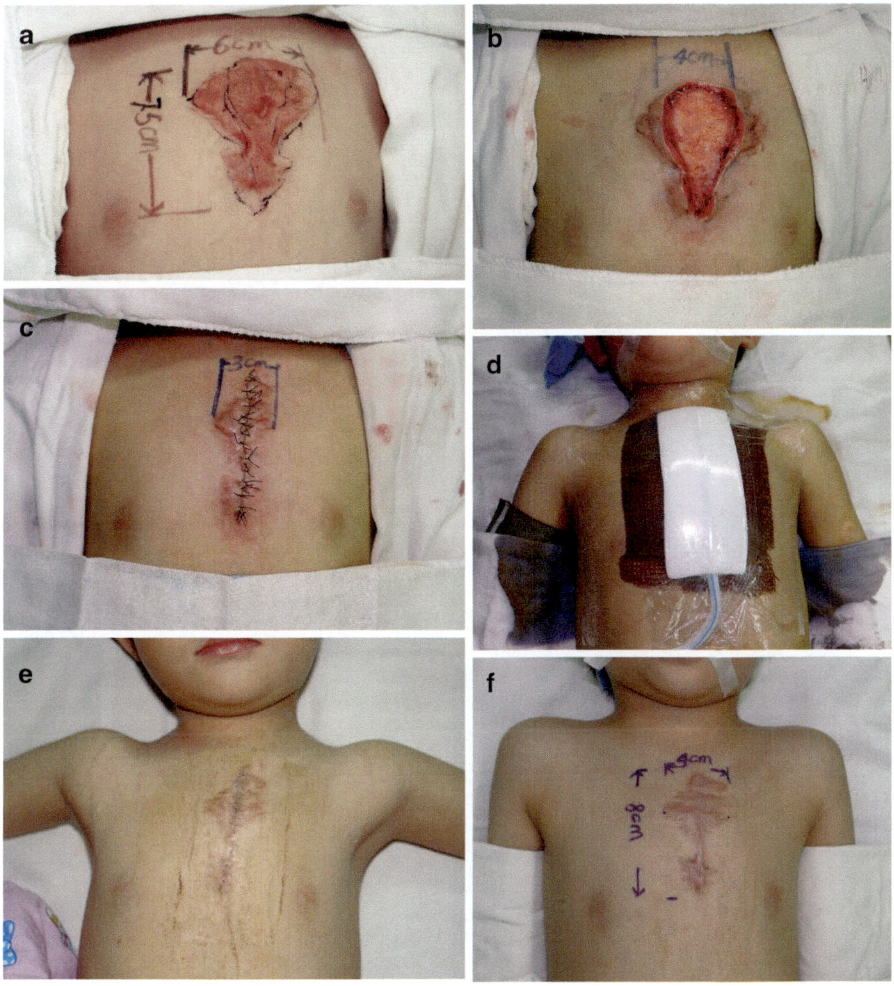

Fig. 7.16 Staged scar excision combined with NPWT technique to treat hypertrophic scar in the chest of a child. (**a**) Chest scar before the first operation. (**b**) A partial excision was performed. (**c**) Suture of the incision. (**d**) The incision was fixed and drained with NPWT technique. (**e**) The incision healed and the scar was reduced significantly. (**f**) Measurement before the second operation. The scar area was significantly smaller than that in (**a**). (**g**) Obvious tension along the incision after the second operation. (**h**) Suture of the incision. (**i**) The incision was covered and drained with NPWT technique. (**j**) The incision healed and the scar area was significantly smaller than that in (**f**). (**k**) Six months after the second operation, the appearance was significantly improved, with a significantly smaller scar than that in (**a**)

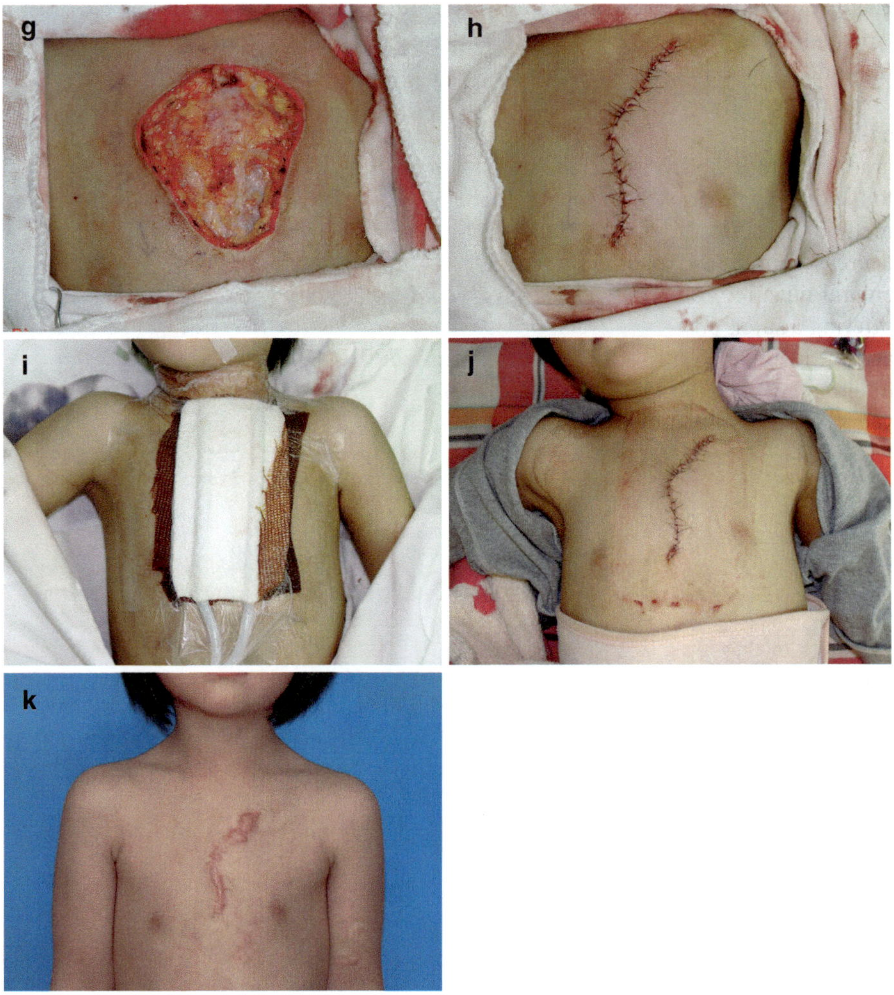

Fig. 7.16 (continued)

associated with larger scar development [14]. Scar revision procedures involving extensive tissue removal inherently introduce increased tension along the incision site, elevating the risk of hypertrophic scar formation. To mitigate this tension, a range of products have been developed to address scar management [15–17]. These products aim to diminish fibrosis at the surgical site, foster tissue regeneration, and notably reduce scar formation. They can be broadly classified into two categories: invasive options such as wound tension reduction devices utilizing skin staplers and noninvasive alternatives like tension-relief tapes or other devices designed for offloading wound tension without invasive measures. However, noninvasive products may encounter issues such as displacement and challenges during dressing changes, while invasive solutions, while effective in reducing tension, may lead to varying degrees of skin trauma from suturing that can impact the cosmetic outcome.

In lieu of the aforementioned approaches, we have incorporated the technique of NPWT [18] into our surgical incision management protocol. It improves healing outcomes by facilitating efficient drainage, secure fixation, and tension alleviation along the incision. The key advantages of NPWT encompass:

① **Tension transfer:** This mechanism involves appropriately loosening the skin on both sides of the incision through a force that brings them toward each other using a sterile film. Consequently, normal skin distant from the incision experiences heightened tension, effectively transferring it away from the incision site.

② **"Suction cup effect" of NPWT:** NPWT creates a seal between the wound bed and the dressing, maintaining a controlled negative pressure environment that tightens the skin and tissue toward the center. This action further diminishes tension along the incision.

③ **"Leveling effect" of negative pressure:** NPWT fosters a more uniform distribution of pressure across the wound surface, reducing localized areas of high pressure and promoting consistent healing throughout the wound bed. This alignment aids in harmonizing uneven scar tissues adjacent to the incision through close adherence to negative pressure materials.

④ **Fluid Management and Circulation Improvement:** NPWT dressing, when applied over a wound, generates negative pressure within the dressing, facilitating drainage of excess fluid, reduction of edema, enhancement of local circulation, and stimulation of granulation tissue formation.

⑤ **Enhanced Suturing and Cosmetic Outcome:** The use of finer sutures for improved cosmetic results becomes feasible with NPWT, allowing for earlier suture removal and thereby reducing the risk of scar hypertrophy.

⑥ **Simplicity and Efficacy:** In comparison to alternative tension reduction methods, this method stands out for its straightforward operation, definitive effectiveness, and absence of associated collateral injuries.

Based on our clinical observations, all patients undergoing scar revision using this method exhibited notable reductions in scar size, thickness, hyperemia, pigmentation, and associated discomfort, leading to a substantial enhancement in overall appearance. Posttreatment POSAS assessments showed improved outcomes. Both patients and their families expressed high levels of satisfaction with the results. Furthermore, some parents reported observing increased liveliness and improved demeanor in their children following the scar revision procedure.

Compared with traditional revision methods using skin grafting or expander, this method offers distinct advantages: ① **Consistent Color Matching:** The surgical incision blends seamlessly with the surrounding skin. ② **No donor site and hence no additional scarring**. ③ **Simplicity and Versatility:** The procedure is straightforward and can be performed across a wide age range without strict limitations. ④ **Minimal Incisions and Reduced Risks:** With fewer cuts and lower potential for collateral damage, this method minimizes the risk of unintended injuries. ⑤**Efficient Tension Reduction and Reliable Fixation:** The technique simplifies tension management without causing additional harm, ensures fixation and secure wound closure.

However, it is important to acknowledge some limitations of this approach. Not all patients are suitable candidates for direct excision, and some individuals may require multiple procedures of this nature, possibly necessitating the use of expanders at a later stage. Despite these considerations, the method remains valuable for its ability to significantly decrease the need for extensive skin grafting and mitigate the complexities associated with expander design and operation.

(Chuanan Shen, Jianhua Cai)

7.2.2 NPWT Following Z-Plasty for Scar Contracture Release

[Background]

Burn patients often experience functional limitations and aesthetic challenges if they develop linear and cord-like or web-shaped contractures. To correct these contractures, Z-plasty procedures involving one or more Z-shaped incisions are commonly employed due to their safety, relative simplicity, and favorable outcomes with a low recurrence rate of contractures [19]. However, in practice, the flaps of the Zs might necrotize due to inadequate blood supply, a common issue associated with traditional suturing and stenting methods. This results in an undermined healing process, which may require prolonged dressing changes or a second surgery of correction. Therefore, it is clinically significant to find effective solutions to minimize the risk of ischemic necrosis of the flaps and optimize the healing process for contracture release [20].

In recent years, we have incorporated NPWT into the management of contracture release and achieved positive clinical outcomes [21].

[Protocol]

I. Indications

Patients with severe contracture who need Z-plasty procedures involving one or several Z-shaped incisions

II. Preoperative preparation

Prior to the procedure, bacterial cultures are obtained from creases in the scar. The patient should have a bath and have the contracture area diligently cleansed before the operation. Standard preoperative tests and assessments are performed, with particular attention given to ensuring well-controlled blood glucose levels in diabetic patients. Effective preoperative communication is maintained, and informed consent is duly obtained from all patients undergoing the procedure.

III. Surgical method

1. **Position of the patient.** The surgical field must be fully exposed for optimal access. In cases where the surgical site is located on the lateral trunk or axilla, a lateral lying position may be adopted.

2. **Surgical site preparation.** Thorough disinfection of the surgical area is carried out using iodine tincture and alcohol before draping. Any folds or hidden cavities within the scar are meticulously cleansed with alcohol-impregnated gauze.
3. **Scar excision and contracture release.** One or more Z-shaped incisions are strategically planned along the linear or cord-like contracture to facilitate release. The limbs of the Zs are transposed to alleviate the tension along the contracture. Attention should be paid to ensure adequate blood supply to the limbs, taking into account their specific types and length-to-width ratios.
4. **Application of NPWT.** A tubeless NPWT system is preferred to deliver the benefits of negative pressure therapy without compromising blood supply to the tips of the limbs. This system avoids the compression from direct contact with drainage tubes in the traditional tubing-based NPWT devices. Once properly positioned, the NPWT system is sealed airtight with a film and secured with outer dressings.

[Typical Case]

The patient, a 46-year-old female, developed multiple scar hyperplasia and contractures following a burn injury. The right axillary contracture severely limited mobility in her right shoulder and right upper limb, allowing only a 60-degree extension. A comprehensive Z-plasty involving five limbs of Zs was meticulously planned to fully release the axillary contracture. The surgical field was continuously treated with a tubeless NPWT system, and the shoulder joint was kept in abduction. Postoperatively, the patient remained stable, with optimal blood supply to the flaps and no signs of ischemic necrosis. The surgical incisions healed smoothly, resulting in an even surface. Notably, there was a marked improvement in the appearance of the right axilla and enhanced functionality of the right shoulder. Ultimately, the right upper extremity achieved a significant increase in extension, reaching 150 degrees upon complete healing (Figs. 7.17, 7.18, 7.19, 7.20, 7.21, and 7.22).

[Discussion]

NPWT serves two crucial functions in wound management. Firstly, it provides physical isolation for the wound through its airtight structure, and secondly, it exerts a biomechanical effect with its sustained suction force [22].

In our experience with NPWT to aid postoperative care of contracture release, we have observed several positive outcomes. These include ensuring robust blood supply to the flaps, absence of complications such as local blisters, epidermal floatation, or necrosis of flap tips, and successful healing of incisions within the flap areas. NPWT also minimizes other potential risks associated with changes in body position [23].

To maximize the benefits of NPWT in contracture release, specific technical considerations are crucial:

① **Maintaining Optimal Negative Pressure:** It is recommended to sustain negative pressure levels between 0.02 and 0.03 MPa.

② **Preference for Tubeless Systems:** Utilizing a tubeless NPWT system is preferred to prevent compression from direct tubing contact with the wound. If

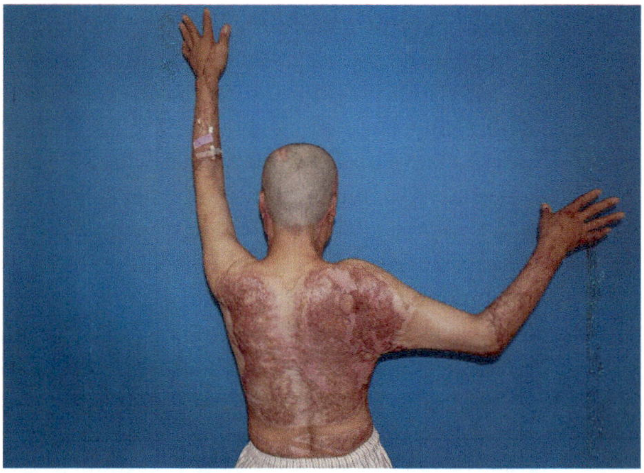

Fig. 7.17 Right axillary contracture

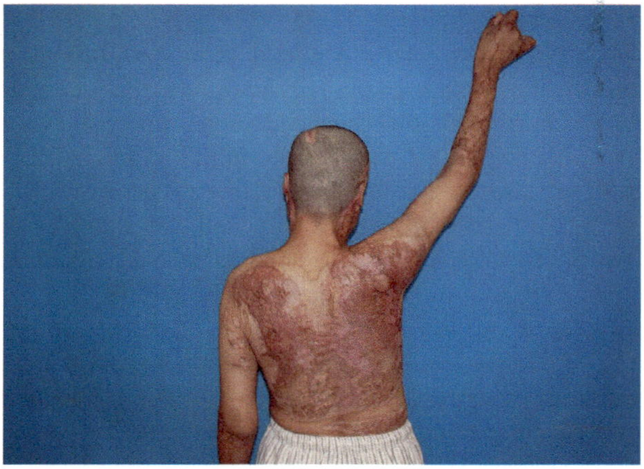

Fig. 7.18 Enhanced functionality of the right axilla and the right upper extremity

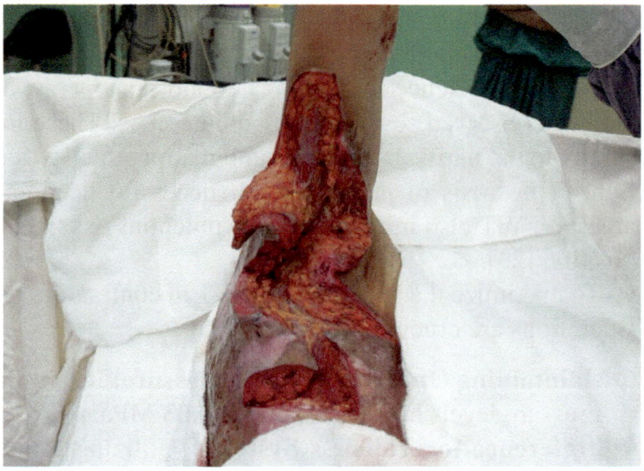

Fig. 7.19 A Z-plasty involving 5 limbs of Zs was performed to release the axillary contracture